FACE MASK

Table of Contents

HOMEMADE MEDICAL FACE MASK PATTERN............ 5

INTRODUCTION 6

CHAPTER 1:WHAT IS A FACE MASK? 7

CHAPTER 2. WHEN TO USE A MASK? 11

Preventing Infection Acquisition:.................................12

CHAPTER 3: HOW TO WEAR A FACE MASK PROPERLY:........................... 15

How to wear a DIY face mask: 19

Filtering respiratory system 22

CHAPTER 4: HOW TO PROPERLY REMOVE YOUR MASK? 25

Uses of a medical face cover 27

CHAPTER 5: ARE MASKS EVEN EFFECTIVE? 29

Are homemade masks effective for healthcare workers? 36

CHAPTER 6: BUILDING AN EFFECTIVE FACE MASK 42

What to do when you don't have sewing materials: 45

CHAPTER 7: WILL HOSPITALS ACCEPT HOMEMADE MASKS? 49

CHAPTER 8: GUIDELINES FOR WEARING A FACE-COVERING................ 53

Why are face masks necessary? 56

CHAPTER 9: HOMEMADE FACE MASK 60

CHAPTER 10: TAKE THE FOLLOWING PRECAUTIONS TO PROTECT YOURSELF:.. 64

Materials 69

CONCLUSION.. 75

DIY REUSABLE FACE MASK PATTERN 76

INTRODUCTION... 77

CHAPTER 1: BEST FACE MASK FOR VIRUS PROTECTION 78

1. Mask respirator 78

2. Face Masks disposable Co-power 79

3. Nuisance dust mask Honeywell, disposable 80

4. Medical Mask 3M N95 1860 82

5. Disposable mask 3layer breathable safety filter 83

6. Dynarex 2201 Medical-surgical face mask 84

7. Folding mask respirator SolidWorks 85

8. Kimberly-Clark mask Fluid Shield Procedure Face 87

9. 4530 universal heavy-duty non-toxic safety masks 88

10. Ellipse GVS SPR451 P100 Half respiratory mask 89

CHAPTER 2: EXAMPLE OF FACE MASK PATTERN 90

Material required for the first method 92

Disposables 94

CHAPTER 3: SOME ADVICE BEFORE YOU GET STARTED 96

I put in strong guard before spending time sewing masks: 99

CHAPTER 4: THE BEST MATERIALS TO MAKE A FACE MASK 100

For fabric loops, if you are not using elastic: **102**

And if you cannot find elastic? 106

CHAPTER 5: HOW IS A CLOTH MASK USED? 110

Recommended products 112

Explanation 114

N95 masks must be appropriately fitted to work effectively **119**

CHAPTER 6: PROBLEMS WITH A HOMEMADE MASK 123

Many risks associated with cloth masks 125

CHAPTER 7: WHY DO YOU NEED A FACE MASK FOR PROTECTION ANTIVIRUS? 131

CHAPTER 8: THERE IS ALSO THE N95 MASKS OR REUSABLE P100 134

CONCLUSION 137

DIY HOMEMADE MEDICAL FACE MASK **138**

INTRODUCTION 139

CHAPTER 1: 7 WAYS TO MAKE A CREATIVE FACE MASK 140

1. **HOW TO MAKE A FACE MASK WITH A SOCK**.............................140

2. **MAKING A FACE MASK WITH AN OLD T-SHIRT** 141

3. **HOW TO MAKE A FACE MASK WITH A HANDKERCHIEF** 142

4. **HOW TO MAKE A FACE MASK WITH A SCARF INFINITY**..............143

5. **HOW TO MAKE A FACE MASK WITH A BUFF** 143

6. **MAKING A MASK AND HEADBAND COMBO** 144

7. **HOW TO MAKE A FACE MASK WITH SEWING MACHINE** 145

CHAPTER 2: THE REASON WHY THE FACE MASK IS A SOCIAL BOOST147

CHAPTER 3: COVID-19 IMPACT ON THE WORLD ECONOMY 153

Efforts and resources of the State Department 158

CHAPTER 4: OUR GLOBAL HEALTH LEADERSHIP 161

Building Global Health Security for the first line 164

CHAPTER 5: WHAT IS THE IMPACT OF CORONAVIRUS ON ECONOMY?
.... 168

Coronavirus has little impact on the confidence of European business. 170

CHAPTER 6: THE IMPACT OF COVID-19 HAD ON TOURISM. 172

The SARS coronavirus has killed nearly 800 people then. 179

T'Way launch air is stopped due to virus concerns. 183

CHAPTER 7: HOW TO THINK OF TRAVEL AS IT EVOLVES THE CORONAVIRUS THREAT 187

CHAPTER 8: THESE AIRLINES OFFER FLEXIBLE TRAVEL OPTIONS, ADAPT TO THE SPREAD OF THE CORONA. 190

CHAPTER 9: WHAT YOU NEED TO KNOW ABOUT CORONAVIRUSES .. 193

Economic forecasts.. 199

CONCLUSION 216

HOMEMADE MEDICAL FACE MASK PATTERN

INTRODUCTION

This book is all about the type of generally made mask, and use is likely to decrease viral exposure and infection risk on a population level, despite poor and imperfect adherence, personal respirators providing most protection. Masks worn by patients may not offer as high a degree of protection against aerosol transmission.

CHAPTER 1: WHAT IS A FACE MASK?

Face masks are a medical device used to prevent and reduce the risk of spreading infectious diseases. It can also be recognized as isolation, laser, dental, procedural, medical, the face masks are significant to ensure an excellent adequate and safe coverage of the nose and mouth, and have earrings or ties or bands in the back of the head. There are many models on the market, different in use, context, originality, and available in various colours. It is essential for using an FDA approved face mask.

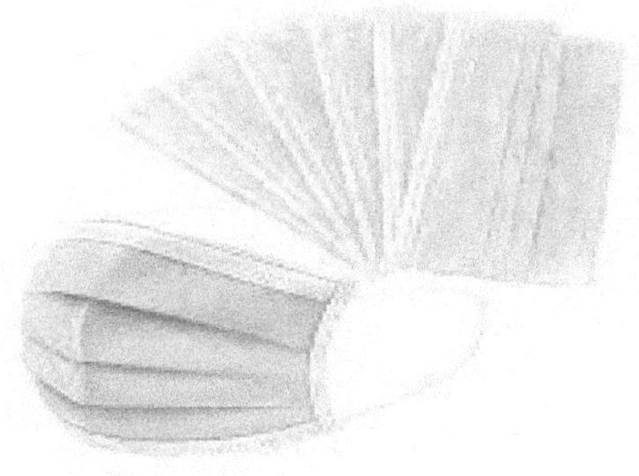

What is the use of a face mask?

Facemasks of sneezing or sprays of coughs, or other body help limit the spread of germs and bacteria. When someone talks, coughs or sneezes, they can release tiny drops of saliva into the air, that can infect others. When someone is sick, a face mask can limit the number of germs and bacteria, which would otherwise be released to the outside by breathing. So, whoever wears the cover can protect himself and other people from the risk of bacteriological contagion. Pay attention to correctly using a face mask to ensure adequate protection of the wearer' swearer's respiratory tract, so as not to come into direct contact with splashes fluids.

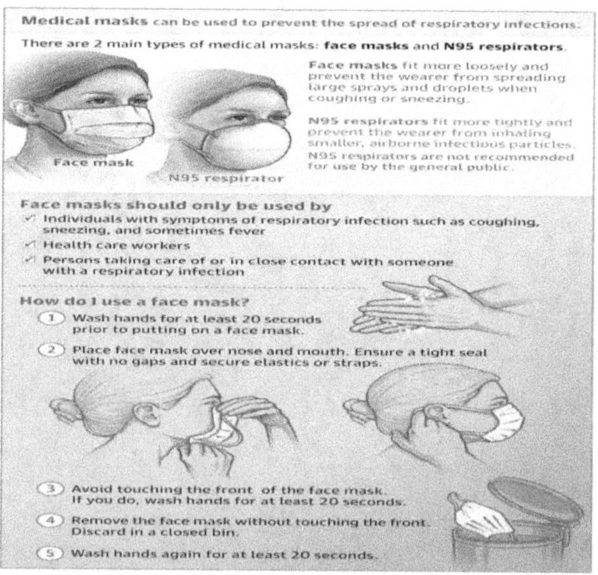

When to wear a face mask correctly?

Keep in mind that in case you are sick with cough or sneeze (with or without fever) and you know you need to get in touch together other people. Wearing the mask will help protect them from catching the disease, or spread it further in case you already have it. Healthcare settings have imposed specific rules for when people should wear face masks.

Medical masks are a Signiant medical aid, that can be used to prevent and avoid infections, which can cause respiratory problems.

This type of personal protective equipment is used to prevent the spread of respiratory infections and spread a potentially lethal virus for humanity like wildfire. These masks cover the wearer' swearer's mouth and nose and, if worn correctly, can be useful in preventing the transmission of respiratory viruses and bacteria.

There are two main models of masks considered Signiant and used against viral diseases, the prevention of respiratory infections, the so-called surgical masks, which are classed into facial and respiratory masks.

These masks differ according to the type of use for which they are intended and according to the size of infectious particles that manage to filter, and therefore not to pass. Face masks are usually suitable for viruses that cause damage to the respiratory tract. For this reason, they are particularly suitable and produced so as not to allow the transmission of these viruses, through the droplets produced by a sneeze, a cough, or even an animated discussion in tight and closed environments, where they travel short distances but are highly contagious. A classic example is the n95 respirators, which take their name from the characteristic of how they are made. They prevent access to the airways of 95% of light airborne particles. They are constructed to be perfectly adherent to the face, so as not to allow the inhalation of smaller infectious particles that can spread in the air over medium-long distances, through coughing and sneezing. There are some diseases where the use of N95 respirators is crucial. Among these diseases, the most common are tuberculosis, chickenpox, and measles. It should also be considered that for appropriate use of these particular N95 respirators must be carried out on individuals who do not have facial hair.

CHAPTER 2. WHEN TO USE A MASK?

Face masks should not be used only by people who have symptoms such as coughing, sneezing, or, in some cases, fever. Face masks should be worn primarily by healthcare professionals and by people who care for or are in close contact with patients with respiratory infections. By now we have reached the point that they must also be worn by healthy individuals to protect themselves from the acquisition of respiratory diseases because it is possible to come into contact with the so-called asymptomatic, or people who have not developed any symptoms but are healthy carriers, and a vehicle for the transmission of the virologic infection. When requests for masks intensify, to cope with emergencies, they should be reserved for those who need them most because coverages can be scarce during periods of diffuse respiratory infection. Therefore, a limited presence of masks may occur sold on the market. Because N95 respirators require specialized t testing, they are not recommended for use by the general public.

Preventing Infection Acquisition:

The perfect way to prevent the acquisition and spread of respiratory infections is to apply proper hand hygiene. Wash your hands often. Good advice suggests that you avoid touching difficult parts of disease, such as the nose, eyes, or mouth, before adequately cleaning and disinfecting your hands. Avoid close contact with other patients. Besides, appropriate cleaning of surfaces and domestic environments using special sanitizers, such as wipes or cleaning sprays.

How to wear a face mask

First of all, clean your hands with soap and water or use hand sanitizer before touching the mask.

Take off a mask from the box and make sure there are no visible tears or holes in either side of the cover.

Determine which right side of the mask is the top.

Front of the cover, which has a rigid edge bent over and intended to mould to the shape of your nose.

Determine which right side of the mask is the front.

The coloured side of the cover is usually the front and should face away from you, while the white hand touches your face.

Follow the instructions below, paying attention to the type of mask you are using.

- Face Mask with Ear-loops:
- Hold the mask by the ear loops.
- Place a circle around each ear.

Face Mask with Ties:

Carry the mask to the nose level and place the ties over the crown of the head, and secure with a bow.

Face Mask with Bands:

Hold the mask in hand with the nosepiece or top of the costume at undertips, making sure that the headbands are hung under the palms.

Carry the cover to the nose level and pull the upper strap over the head, until it sits on top of the head.

Pull the lower strap over until it rests on the nape of the neck.

Mould or pinch the hard edge to the shape of the nose. In case you are using a face mask with ties:

Then take the bottom links, one in each hand, and secure them, making a bow at the nape of the neck.

How to take off a face mask

First of all, clean your hands with soap and water or hand sanitizer before touching the mask. Avoid touching the front of the cover. The front of the hood is contaminated. Only contact the ear loops/ties/band.

How to put on a Mask

If it is required to wear a mask, it is a vital measure to sanitize the hands, mixing soap and water, and rinsing for 30 seconds, and then you can safely use it. An excellent solution sees the use of an alcohol-based disinfectant, the content of which must be at least 60% alcohol.

This method can also replace or be complementary to washing with soap and water.

After cleaning the hands, place the face mask over the nose and the mouth. Be sure to ensure an airtight seal with your face. When you are wearing the mask, do not touch it, to leave it as hygienic as possible If you do feel the face mask, wash your hands, or use hand sanitizer again. After using it, remove it without touching the front of the face mask and throw it in the trash, without letting it come into contact with objects or people. Rewash your hands after dropping the face masks.

CHAPTER 3: HOW TO WEAR A FACE MASK PROPERLY:

Likely, you've never had to worry about adequately covering your nose and mouth before you and yourself being a patient in the hospital or working in medicine or construction. With the intersection of the risk of infection, surgical face masks, as well as face cloth coverings, both those purchased online and those created at home, are acquiring greater relevance and importance in the world. They are becoming a necessity during the novel coronavirus pandemic that has affected Americans in all 50 states, and the whole world.

Experts for Disease Control and Prevention are advising everyone wears face coverings in public and leaders in communities, and single states can also be mandating that you do so.

In the last period, New York Governor Andrew Cuomo approved a new legislature asking citizens to put on a face mask when social distancing measures aren't possible, including those activities with a high risk of close contacts, such as taking a means of public transport or those essential businesses in enclosed spaces. Same shortly after that, leaders in Southern California passed similar guidelines with more donate recommendations for essential workers with increased risk of closed contact.

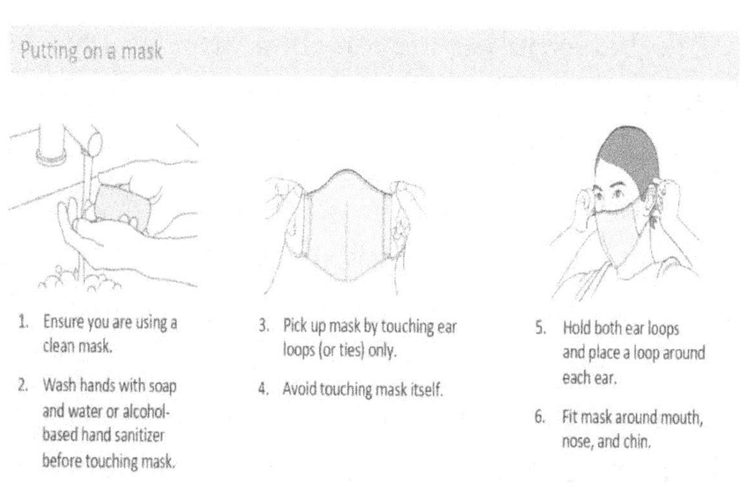

The correct way to wear a medical or homemade mask:

Bring up your mask by its ear loops. Without touching the cover, itself, bring the circuits up to your ears, securing them as tightly as possible. If the hood is equipped with ties instead of loops, tie the top pair around the lower crown of your head, and the second pair around the nape of the neck.

Be careful that it covers the nose and the mouth. The mask hinders the external emission of bacteria into the air by covering nose and mouth, wearing a medical mask correctly, it can also provide slight protection, and increase your chances of repelling any nearby particles and germs.

The mask must be adjusted so that it adheres perfectly and covers the chin, lifting it to the base of the jaw. Pulling the hood under the button is a surer way not always to have to adjust it when you leave the house, Secure the mask around the bridge of the nose. Some covers are equipped with a metal tab to be positioned at the trunk (in fact, if you feel a metal tab on the chin, you will know that the cover has been placed upside down). Make sure that the top of the mask is snug against your face. In case there is no metal tongue, make sure it doesn't slip off your nose afterwards.

While surgical masks are unable to filter all the particles and bacteria present in the air, the N95 covers are also used by healthcare professionals, so there is no need to worry about the filtering, which is guaranteed. In this case, you will only have to provide full adherence to the face to obtain effective screening.

MASK INSTRUCTIONS
IT'S BETTER TO USE THE RIGHT WAY TO WEAR

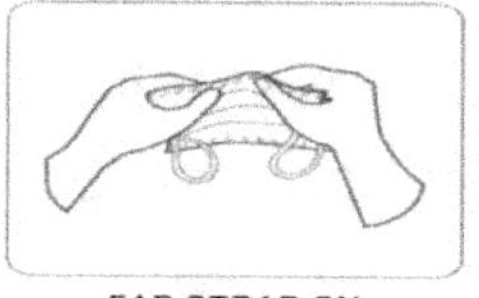

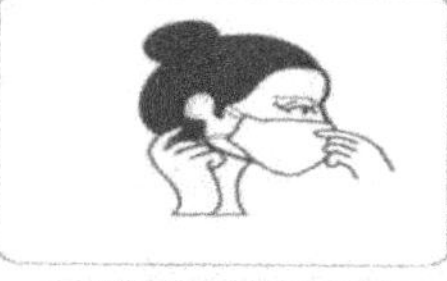

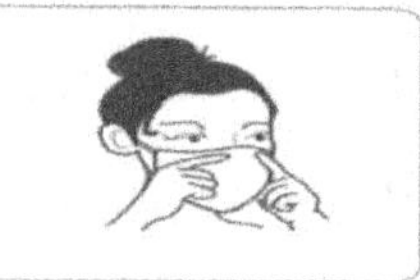

MATTERS NEEDING ATTENTION

1. THE MASK SHOULD BE REPLACED IN TIME, NOT RECOMMENDED FOR LONG-TERM USE
2. IT IS RECOMMENDED TO STOP USING IF THERE IS ANY MALADJUSTMENT OR ADVERSE REACTION DURING WEARING
3. THIS PRODUCT IS NOT WASHABLE, PLEASE MAKE SURE IT IS USED WITHIN THE VALIDITY PERIOD
4. STORE IN A DRY AND VENTILATED PLACE AWAY FROM FIRE ANDINFLAMMABLES

How to recognize the external side of a surgical mask?

If you have a medical-grade surgical mask, you may be wondering which side should be on the outside. Although not all manufacturers follow the same style and therefore, not all products are built in the same way, according to expert opinion, in traditional models, usually, the coloured part of the mask represents the outer side. According to Dr Rohede's view: "Looking carefully at the mask, you can consider dividing it into an "internal" and an "external" side, to understand which part should be put on the face." He also explains:

"For most surgical masks I have worn while working in public health, the colouring is turned outward."

How to wear a DIY face mask:

If you don't have a surgical mask or a hand-sewn mask, using a cloth face covering will still prevent you from spreading bacteria through droplets in public places." Dr Bearman says. "None of the masks is medical-grade, and any gaps are less important, as these are meant to prevent droplets and not aerosols. It has been widely demonstrated how COVID-19 manages to transmit through larger particles inside droplets and not through aerosols in everyday spaces, outside hospitals." Plus, a face-covering might act as a human "dog cone" in that it reminds you to avoid touching your face.

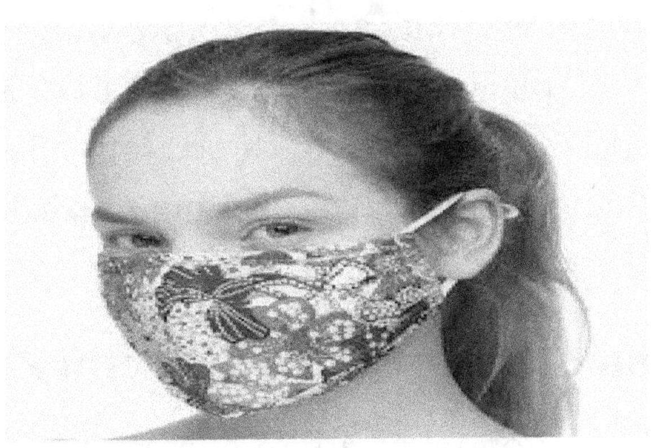

How can I clean my mask properly?

After safely removing the mask or linings by handling its ties or loops with care, Dr Bearman says that any surgical masks should be disposed of, as these are for single use only. Experts say it is wrong to attempt to disinfect surgical masks at home, although some health professionals may do it due to a shortage of supplies, all experts do not recommend doing it at home. There isn't any actual data on how you should washcloth coverings. Still, Carolyn Forte, Director of the Good Housekeeping Institute Cleaning Lab, suggests washing each mask, using hot water in washing machines, and drying in a dryer at warm temperatures.

When you intend to keep the fabric covering at home, before washing it, you should put it in a dry paper bag. According to Dr Bearman's claims, it should be ensured that any moisture contained in the masks must dry out, and therefore may not dry out properly if placed in a closed box. Dr Rohde adds that it's best to have two or three cloth masks that you can cycle between to avoid having to wash your cloth mask every time you head outside.

When and how to wear medical masks

When you take care of someone with the virus,

you must take the necessary safety measures and wear a mask.

Wear a mask when you are coughing or sneezing.

Masks are a useful prevention tool, only if combined with frequent hand cleaning, rubbing it with alcohol or soap and water.

When you wear a mask, you also need to know the method on how to use it and dispose of it properly.

What to know about mask protection?

A protective mask is a device intended to protect the user from inhalation of harmful dust, pathogens, fumes, vapours, or gases. The covers and application in different sectors of use, from the military ones, from the private sector, and the public, they range from the cheapest, single-use, reusable disposable masks to replaceable cartridge models.

There are two categories of breathing apparatus, namely "filtering" device, which can be either passive or active and which force contaminated air to pass through a filtering element, and "insulating" apparatus, in which fresh air is delivered from a reserve. Within each category, different techniques are used to reduce or eliminate the harmful airborne matter. History of the development of protective

Masks intended to protect against the inhalation of particles have probably been around for a long time for mining or dust sources. During epidemics of plagues, the doctors being made masks in the beak of birds called with medicinal plants supposed to kill the miasmas responsible for the contagion; In the middle of the xix the century, medical masks appear.

During the XX century, during the origins of the tanks, their occupants (pilot, gunner) were forced to wear a mask to protect themselves from the fragments of paint and metal ejected from the walls by the impacts of projectiles to the outside.

Metal protective helmets/masks with a window for vision are currently only used in metallurgy and for welding and tend to be replaced by masks made of lighter composite materials. For uses without a heat source, the plexiglass in thick sheet (1 to 5 mm) is transparent and impact resistant. Sometimes, a genuine visor made of a flexible and transparent plastic protects the face of the operator from splashes of corrosive liquid or at toxic, biological or medical risks (splashes of droplets, blood, etc.

Filtering respiratory system

Wool filter masks were used by early inventors such as Haslett and Tyndall. Wool is still used as a filter today. Wool filter masks were used by first inventors such as Haslett and Tyndall. Today wool is still used as a filter, together with other substances such as glass, cellulose, plastic, and combinations of two or more of these materials. Since filters cannot be cleaned and reused and therefore have a limited lifespan, costs and availability are key factors. There are disposable and cartridge models. Since filters cannot be cleaned and reused and therefore have a limited lifespan, price and availability are key factors. There are disposable models, as well as cartridge models.

How to put on a general public mask and wear it?

First, let's remember a few instructions: the little ones should not wear a mask.

For children under 3, wearing a mask is therefore

prohibited due to the risk of suffocation. The second important point, the cover is not a spacesuit; it does not protect itself from the virus and should not be seen as a free passport.

Its port must be accompanied by respect and the practice of barrier gestures.

For a mask, whether surgical or fabric, to be effective, you still have to put it on!

Several steps are to be followed carefully.

Wash the hands before putting on your mask to avoid risking soiling immediately.

Always grab it by the elastic bands to position it.

Place it well by checking in front of a mirror that covers all the essential areas: nose, mouth, but also chin.

Upon express request of the organizing committee for the Paris 2024 Olympic Games, several champions carried out video demonstrations. Here is one featuring via-time Olympic biathlon champion Martin Fourcade.

CHAPTER 4: HOW TO PROPERLY REMOVE YOUR MASK?

The steps to follow

- ➢ small freezer bag, etc.;) Have you finished your outing, or need to replace your mask for another after 4hours? Removing your cover must also obey specifics rules.
- ➢ Handle the mask only with rubber bands and remember that the outside of the cover can be potentially soiled and infected.
- ➢ Place it in an airtight box if possible while waiting for a wash.
- ➢ Wash your hands immediately.
- ➢ When it is a disposable mask, throw it away immediately, preferably in a closed bin, and, if possible, in an airtight bag in which you enclose your cover.

Washing your mask: tips and mistakes to avoid

Once your mask has been removed, it should still be washed before each new use. To clean your cover, you must comply with strict health regulations.

First of all, remember that it is imperative to wash it after each use, has provided recommendations plug.

The washing of the general public fabric mask must be done in the washing machine via a cycle of a minimum of 30 minutes at 60 degrees. A scientifically validated process kills all bacteria.

First, remember to clean your washing machine, especially with bleach, to keep your drum clean. You can also spin it vacuum once at 60 degrees to kill any bacteria.

Place your masks in the drum, best to wash them separately from the rest of your laundry. You can, however, place them with old sheets if you have to clean them. If you want to spin linen with 60 degrees, you can put your masks in a dedicated bag (for example, those for lingerie).

Once the laundry is done, take out your masks and put them to dry. They must be dry after two hours of drying. If this is not the case and if you do not have a dryer, you can speed up the drying with a hairdryer.

To end out everything and avoid making mistakes regarding the maintenance of your general public mask, you can end what you are looking for in our dedicated le.

Uses of a medical face cover

The environmental protection by contaminated droplets from the potentially infected wearer, particularly in medicine and caretaking.

Protection of wearer from splashes of infectious bodily fluids, e.g., during surgery. (With appropriate additional application) Restricted protection of wearer from smear infection from unclean hands touching the mouth and nose.

What protection does the mask offer?

Most experts estimate that wearing mouth-nose protection reduces the risk of infection for other people because it captures to a specie extent droplet during talking, sneezing, or coughing. However, natural masks are not able on their own to perform efficient protection if the wearer s infected with the coronavirus. But there are also side effects. Wearing masks could ensure that people kept more distance from each other.

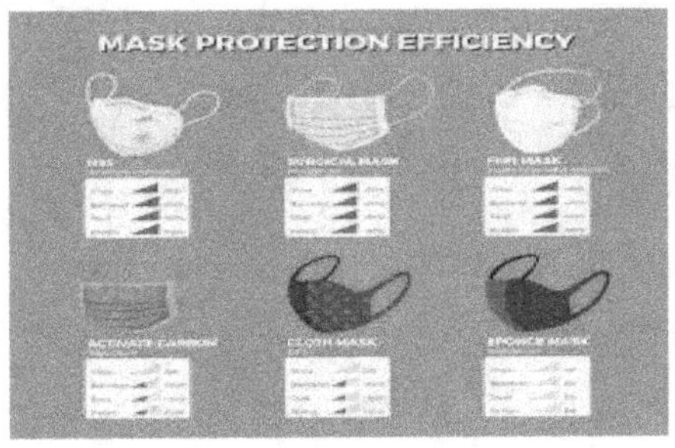

In what situations is it advisable to wear a mask?

Its recommended to wear everyday masks in public life - especially when shopping as well as on the bus and train. If a safety distance of at least 1.5 meters can be maintained or if there is alternative protection, for example, at the supermarket checkout - for instance, in partitions - then it is not necessary to wear masks.

How do I wear it?

- Masks are only useful if you wear them correctly. The WHO (World Health Organization) has provided some essential instructions:
- Wash the hands at least for 20 seconds, using water mixed with soap before touching or wearing the mask.
- Ensure that your nose and mouth are completely covered when you wear it.
- Do not touch the mask while you are out, this in order not to contaminate it.
- Do not take off the mask while 'you're in public.
- To remove the mask once you return, untie it from the back. Don't touch the front of it.

- First of all, after returning home, you immediately wash the mask, so it doesn't contaminate your things.
- Wash your hands continuously, both immediately before putting it on and after removing it, and repeat the procedure even when you are wearing a new mask.

-

CHAPTER 5: ARE MASKS EVEN EFFECTIVE?

Some studies on homemade masks have shown that they are less effective than surgical masks and certainly cannot replace or compete for efficacy, with the first N95 respirators that health workers, who were wearing them, allow them to treat patients and take lesser risks.

Dr Koushik an internal physician, residing at the Johns Hopkins Bayview Medical Center in Maryland, says: "Homemade masks are partially effective."

They also make it possible to get a physical barrier and defend against infective particles, he said, they don't have a sound alteration system and filters as effective as those used by N95 respirators.

But compared to nothing, it is always better to have

them, especially useful for those who leave the house to make a quick trip to the grocery or pharmacy, said Anna Davies and Raina MacIntyre, skilled public health researchers and authors of two separate studies on the effectiveness of cloth masks.

We need to keep in mind that masks are not able to replace the measures of social estrangement that must always exist. First, you need to keep at least six feet apart and stay home as much as possible, as this is still the best way to prevent the virus from spreading.

How do you clean them?

First, you should wash the masks both before and after each use to remove traces of any germs that you may have collected along the way. A washing method is to add the covers in a mesh washing bag and put them to wash in a washing machine so that they do not take off during washing at high temperatures, or decide to remove them directly by hand.

What if I can't make my own?

Crafters on Etsy aren't sold out with masks yet. It is difficult to understand how effective these masks are since you didn't create them yourself, but you can easily compare them with our tutorial on costumes to get an idea of what you want and then buy it: does it cover the nose and mouth? Are there folds?

Will it seal tightly around your face?

It is not necessary to purchase too many masks, given that doctors and prevention experts recommend that only one person per family be assigned to do chores and errands outside the home.

Remember that given the situation, the shipment of masks may take longer than usual, so be careful when purchasing.

Make sure you always wash your masks before putting them on.

In case you can get the masks, keep washing your hands, maintaining measures of social distancing.

Remember, staying at home is the best defence against coronavirus.

It should also be noted and taken into consideration:

Although the situation has worsened in many countries, that of putting on a face cover is advice but not an obligation.

The homemade masks do not, in any way, replace the practices of social estrangement to be adopted together with permanence in one'sone's own homes.

Despite everything, if you need to make a mask, here are some simple detailed instruction, provided by the Centers for the control and prevention of diseases, on the methods to create various models of covers, whether you know how to sew or not.

Necessary materials you'll need to make:

- Bandana, T-shirt or square cotton cloth, about 20" x 20."
- Coffee filter
- Rubber bands or hair ties

How to Make your mask

- For the screen of the mask, you'll need to cut the bottom of a folded coffee filter and keep the top.
- Start to lay a bandana or 20" x 20" T-shirt in a rectangle. Then, fold the bandana or shirt in half lengthwise.
- Then, fold the cut filter in the centre of the folded bandana or shirt.
- Now, fold the top of the bandana or shirt down over the screen. Fold the bottom up.

- In this way, place rubber bands or hair ties around the folded bandana or shirt, about 6 inches apart.
- Then fold the side of the bandana or shirt in toward the middle and tuck.
- Finally, place the rubber bands or hair ties around your ears, and voila, you've made a face mask, no sewing required.

How to sew your mask?

These are the materials you will need to get started: Tightly woven cotton fabric, to prevent germs and other impurities that are found in the air from passing through. Elastics pattern (or rubber bands, string, cloth strips, hair ties), to ensure an effective sewing system on the face.

Needle and thread (or a bobby pin, a sewing machine), scissors. All necessary tools for the correct assembly of the template.

Make your mask

➢ Start to cut your fabric into two 10" by 6" rectangles. Place them on top of each other.
➢ Then, fold over the long sides -- 1/4 inch -- and hem.

- ➤ Now, fold the double layer of fabric over 1/2 inch along the short sides. Stitch down.
- ➤ Thread a 6-inch-long, 1/8-inch-wide piece of elastic through the full hem on each side of the mask and knot it, and this is one of your two ear loops. In case you do not have the elastic, you can use hair ties or rubber bands as an alternative material. In case you only have string or fabric, you can make the relationship longer and tie the mask behind your head. Pull-on the ear loops, so the knots are tucked inside the hem.
- ➤ At this point, you have to collect the sides of the mask on the elastic and adjust it so that the cover to your face.
- ➤ Now, stitch the elastic (or fabric) in place on the corner of the mask to keep it from slipping -- and voila! You'veYou've seen a cover in six steps.

How effective are they?

The health department has determined that homemade fabric masks are not to be considered as valid and adequate personal protective equipment. (PPE) "However, homemade masks can be considered to all intents and purposes, an effective complementary tool to other various methods such as hand washing, social distancing, and other measures aimed at preventing respiratory infections."

"I think it's mostly that people might not become complacent, that they have a homemade mask on.

Fleece said: "Depending on what material they are made of, they can approach the effectiveness of disposable surgical masks."

"But in case you are not using the right material and practising excellent hygiene. "These efforts do nothing but have the negative potential to worsen the situation, providing a false sense of protection in people."

In addition to inappropriate filtering of particles and germs, some masks can also pose additional risks, mostly if we're reusing them. A critical 2015 study published in the medical journal "BMJ OPEN" highlights the risk deriving from the improper use of fabric masks, highlighting how some parameters such as:

"the presence and retention of humidity, inadequate reuse, and imperfect alteration can Significantly affect the increased risk of infection."

So, to use them safely, it is appropriate to use them with logic, awareness, and responsibility, to try to create a sort of barrier between the sick and the healthy.

Is there a way to make better masks?

An influential 2013 study performed by the University of Cambridge states that " the type of material used for homemade masks can have an influential impact on their effectiveness." Also, according to the data analyzed by the same study, some materials are to be considered valid options for the production of a mask, thanks to their ability to help block and filter some virus particles from infected people. Among these articles we need: cotton blend shirts and antimicrobial pillowcases, kitchen tea towels and vacuum cleaner bags

Are homemade masks effective for healthcare workers?

Levine said in a press conference that: "Compared to N95 respirators, or surgical masks, fabric masks are less effective, but they may be better than nothing.

He also acknowledges their inadequacy if provided to healthcare professionals." Naturally, he points out that the fabric masks are not right to use and give to the medical staff employed in the treatment of patients with COVID-19.

According to the words of Ashish K. Jha, the top representative of the Harvard Global Health Institute, the medical community accepted with irony and mockery the recommendation on the use of the bandana by the CDO. Always what Jha said:

"In the presence of a potentially lethal and infected droplet, no evidence has been found that makes the bandana a valid method to protect the doctors and that therefore, in general, it is necessary to protect them with adequate medical protection."

Concerning homemade masks, the CDC also expressed its opinion, not considering them as proper personal protective equipment, as the effectiveness is unknown and is not well established by any evidence. If this decency continues, this will have an impact on healthcare workers, who would thus have few alternatives.

In that case, other options would be considered, which at that point would become necessary.

According to chief medical information offer at Temple University Hospital, David Fleece, "if nothing changes, and there are still evident difficulties in finding the masks, in a short time we will and ourselves without supplies equipment for protection from virologic infections, from which to draw."

According to Fleece, therefore, if nothing should change on the offer side, that of the hand-sewn mask, which is now considered only as an alternative, over time, it could take on greater prominence and be more used.

Can hospitals accept donated masks?

Following the worsening health situation, some hospitals have decided to accept donations of homemade cloth masks.

Still, however, these are sporadic cases, so, before producing a batch of masks to be donated to hospitals, it is advisable to inquire through the local medical facility, if they eventually accept donations.

A striking example was when the Philadelphia Emergency Management Office placed an announcement highlighting the call for help to address the urgent need for surgical masks, especially medical that are not made at home.

Penn Medicine and Jefferson Health are also not accepting homemade mask donations, excluding at least provisionally the acceptance of voluntary contributions of masks sewn at home.

Meanwhile, some organizations, among which the names of Masks for Heroes, and Masks for Docs in Indiana, are proceeding to directly connect the producers and suppliers of masks, with the operators and health institutions that request and accept donations, such as Sew Face Masks Philadelphia.

Whether you are a supplier or a requester, this section is dedicated to those interested in creating or receiving masks, who can check the database to forms to provide or receive covers via the websites of these groups. Preferential in delivering or receiving facial masks.

Always Fleece says that one of the structures in the Philadelphia area, belonging to the health system of Temple University, accepting any donations of do-it-yourself masks. Although evaluation plans have not yet been put in place as to whether and how these donations will be used Currently, Temple Health is corned among the health bodies registered with Mask for Heroes, to facilitate the mask donation procedures that the latter makes available to health bodies. Another institution who said he agreed on future donations of homemade masks, if necessary, was the Philadelphia Children's Hospital, which welcomes new announcing for interested persons to make donations mentioned above, sending them into the structure (3401 Civic Center Boulevard) or let them directly in the main lobby of the hospital itself.

Also, in Fleece's opinion, there is a good chance that homemade masks should also be used, in case the supply of protective devices should continue on this path.

Should I wash my mask?

According to Nate Wardle, the press secretary of the Pennsylvania Department of Health, using detergent and hot water is the most effective method for proper washing of homemade masks. While to dry them, it would be necessary to use techniques that provide drying at high temperatures, to kill all germs and bacteria.

What type of ties do you want?

There are currently several ways to tie a mask to the face, but three main ways will be explained, planned, and illustrated here.

The ties that go around your ears. These are loose ties

that you tie together behind your ears each time you put the mask on. This is simplest to make and requires the least work upfront, but you'll need to tie the cover each time you wear it. You can merely slip it on.

Ear-loops. Elastic may be better than fabric for this style since you'll need the ties to be short and tight enough to stay securely wrapped around your ears, but not so quick and close that they pop off.

The ties that go around the back of the head. You'll want the relationship to be long enough to go around the end of the head horizontally, but short enough that the t won't be too loose.

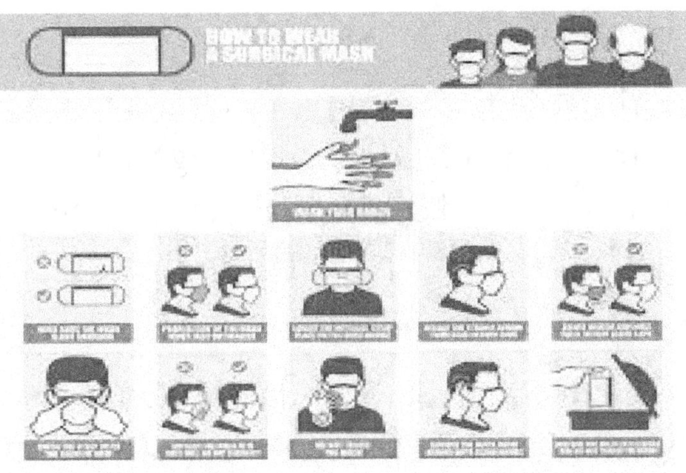

CHAPTER 6: BUILDING AN EFFECTIVE FACE MASK

First Step: Cut two pieces of fabric You want two rectangles, 12 inches wide, and six inches tall Our template is already the right size, so you can just cut out our model, then cut the fabric to t.

Second Step: Sew the fabric rectangles together

Sew the pieces together as tightly as possible. Go along all four sides, about 1/4" to 1/2" from the edge.

Using the template: Place the model on top of the two pieces of fabric and sew all three layers together along the dotted line.

Third Step: Cut fabric or elastic ties. Cut the links to the right size. If you're using fabric ties, you may want to cut wide strips that you can then fold in to hem. That would help keep them from fraying and falling apart when washed.

Fourth Step: Sew the fabric ties to the mask Tightly sew the ends of the fabric ties to the corners of the cover. On the template, sew the links to the marked boxes. For ear loops, create one loop on the left and another on the right, attaching one end at the top of the mask and one end at the bottom.

The forties that go around the back of your head sew each of the four ties to different corners, long enough so that you can tie them behind your head when you put the mask on.

The forties that connect behind your ears, simply sew each of the four ties to different corners.

Fifth Step: Sew around the entire edge again.

Do another pass around the entire outer edge of the mask, ensuring a tight seal between the two pieces of fabric and also securing the ties even further. On the template, sew along the second dotted line.

That's it! Remove the template, if you' you're using it, and your mask is ready to go.

Three ways to upgrade the mask

We have shown you how to make a simple mask, using the advice suggested by the Pennsylvania Department of Health. But, in case, if you have a little more skill and patience, here you can end three exclusive ways with which you can update the mask:

First, let's start by dipping the mask inside-out

instead of leaving the raw edges. In this way, having the frayed edges inside could help keep the cover together and not degrade while being washed. It also looks more beautiful. To do this, the best thing to do will be to sew the ties on one layer, then superimpose the second layer on top of it. At this point, you need to stitch the two layers of fabric together, leaving one or two inches of space instead of completing a complete rectangle. Now, ip the mask inside-out through that rectangle, then sew around the outer edge again.

Fold horizontal pleats. This allows the mask to better the curvature of your face, similar to how surgical masks work. The New York Times has a guide of its own, to make a mask with pleats and that you IP inside-out.

Use the third layer. Some expert seized the opportunity and recommended having two layers of material, but some projects even use a third disposable layer to help better filter the air. Those can include elements that can show them, such as Swiffer disposable dusting pads, coffee filters, paper towels, or something similar. Suzanne Willard, the dean of global health at the Rutgers School of Nursing, says she also uses masks at home using disposable liners.

What to do when you don't have sewing materials:

Remember, homemade masks aren't perfect. So, don't worry about doing everything right as we suggest that the point is to create a crucial mask that covers the nose and mouth, adhering well to the face.

As an alternative method to sewing, you can in case use materials such as safety pins or some clips, to keep the fabric and the bands together. Or staple everything together if necessary.

Don't have the possibility to connect fabric and ties? Don't worry, CDC has non-stitching options in the mask and uses something else. A scarf or bandana can be used if you can make or buy a cover, some tricks to keep in mind about your homemade mask:

First of all, you need to disinfect the mask between every use. The most effective way is to wash it with the rest of the laundry, in hot water and with soap or detergent, then pass it through the dryer and dry in warmer temperatures.

When you are a frequent user, depending on your needs or the type of work and social context you belong to, you may need to create more than one mask, depending on how often you go out.

Take the mask off carefully. Wash your hands before taking the cover off and assume the virus is being collected on the front of the hood. Remember never to touch the front part directly, because the method to remove it properly is with the ties. Remember not to touch your face. Also, wash your hands often even after unmasking.

Masks don't guarantee perfect protection. The use of a cover does not give you the freedom to think of being immune and able to get in touch with others without the risk or otherwise take irresponsible and risky behaviour.

The best behaviour to adapt and continue to stay at home as much as possible and keep the right social distance from others when you leave home.

Is there the best material for a reusable face mask?

However, the best fabric for homemade masks par excellence is a tightly woven, made of 100% cotton fabric. Some interesting ideas for making cotton products is to draw on materials such as sheets, curtains, and woven shirts, considered valid options if they are made entirely of cotton. If you intend to donate the masks, it is highly discouraged the use of knit fabrics (e.g., jersey T-shirts) for the real reason that by stretching, they create holes, which the virus could easily pass. To kill germs and pre-shrink the material, prewash the fabrics with hot water so that it does not change shape after users wash it themselves.

The things you need on top of a sewing machine and fabric are a non-woven interface for reusable masks, intending to block the particles appropriately, then elastic bands or ties to secure it correctly on the face and a piece of metal (like a paperclip) to t it comfortably around the nose without the risk of it slipping away from it. In case you cannot and an interface, you can modify an existing non-woven product, such as HVAC filters or coffee filters, but keep in mind that if you use one of these occasional products, it is better not to use the masks produced as donations if they are not washable. HEPA vacuum bags are also non-woven with functional alteration capabilities; just make them don't contain bar-glass

The beautiful thing about being able to reuse and reinvent products that you already have at home is that you don't have to spend more money to buy them. If you have clothes at home that you no longer use or bed linen, you can very well use them instead of having to buy new fabric. On top of that. All 860 stores offer materials in their classrooms with sewing machines, which, according to the company company's requests, will follow the appropriate recommendations on social distancing. In case you already own a sewing machine, if you prefer not to enter the shop for safety, you can also contact the shop directly, and have the supplies delivered directly outside your car, for a comfortable and safe collection on the sidewalk.

There's also been a buzz around shop towels (usually used by auto mechanics) after a group of seamstresses said they could filter particles better than other at-home face mask materials. As medical laboratories have not yet tested them, they are not however recommended by the CDC, at this point, you can stick with a tightly woven cotton fabric, along with two layers of a non-woven interface. One of the most popular products by women to make a reusable mask is the Hepa vacuum bags.

Young woman with fabric samples for curtains at the table. Multiple colour fabric texture samples selection fabrics for interior decoration. Furniture upholstery

CHAPTER 7: WILL HOSPITALS ACCEPT HOMEMADE MASKS?

Currently, homemade masks are not approved by hospitals, which, with exceptions, will not accept donations of this kind. Check and inquire with the local hospitals in your area if they have provisions to use homemade masks and, if so, what are their procedures they adopt to dispose of them. We must, therefore, consider the rapid evolution of the situation, and the various updates that hospital bodies use to deal with the health emergency.

In unusual cases, if they need it, healthcare professionals are also making requests on social media. There are various portals, which publish these IPR requests from healthcare professionals within social communication channels, such as Instagram pages and groups, Facebook. One of these portals, or Masks for Heroes, which uses an Instagram page to promote IPR requests, and to achieve this goal. To deal with the emergency, some hospitals are said to have given consent to their healthcare workers to send these requests, but with the demand for full anonymity of their identities. There is an institution,

The U.C.

Does it make sense to wear a homemade mouthguard?

Medical protective equipment is urgently needed in nursing and is, unfortunately, also in short supply here. That'sThat's why you see more and more self-made protective masks on the streets and in shops - but do they make any sense, and do they protect the wearer from possible infection? In the following, we explain how the homemade protective masks work and what you should pay attention to.

Does a condent breathing mask protect against infection?

A self-made mouthguard cannot be compared to an FFP2 mask, which protects against aerosols and droplets. A self-made breathing mask does not protect the wearer from infection. However, wearing a makeshift oral and nasal mask can help curb the spread of the coronavirus. Although the cover does not protect the wearer, it serves as a blockage. This means that the wearer of a respirator mask can protect others from infection because pathogens are at least partially retained by the barrier. This is particularly useful if the required distance of two meters cannot be maintained, for example, when shopping.

Necessary: Even if you wear a mask, you should keep your distance, and the hygiene measures (washing and disinfecting hands regularly) take into account.

DIY mouthguard: what should you pay attention to?

It is essential that the mask consists of tightly woven cotton fabric (several layers) and is washed regularly at a minimum of 60 °. It should be cleaned after each wear - so it makes sense to make several masks at once. Please only wear the covers for a short time (e.g., for the time of shopping) and never all day, otherwise incredible viruses can accumulate here. The respirator mask is even safer with an insert that can be replaced (e.g., kitchen paper or hygienic Fleece (e.g., high alteration vacuum cleaner bag, sponge cloth with clean coating, etc.)   see also sewing instructions. Both patterns are designed so that an insert is no problem can be added and exchanged.

Models of protective coatings for the face and face masks:

Currently, there are three main types of protective coatings for the face: fabric, surgical and N95 respirators. Facial fabric coverings are the only coatings that are recommended to wear for the public. While the other models mainly concern health workers.

Fabric face coverings are generally, face coverings, made with household items or made at home with low-cost common materials, which are often already present in our homes.

A cloth face-covering is a facial protective cover to protect and prevent the virus from spreading by moving from those who do not wear it to other healthy people or without symptoms.

Surgical Masks are facial protective covers, typically used in the health sector.

They are used to prevent the risk of infection from infected droplets in the air and ensure protection from all germs except the small particles may carry coronavirus, which, they manage to go beyond them anyway.

N95 Respirator Masks, also called medical respirator

masks, are perfectly tight setting respiratory masks for the face, reserved strictly for health professionals who work in close contact with patients with respiratory infectious diseases and protect them from airborne and fluid hazards. They significantly reduce exposure to particles, including small particle aerosols and large droplets. N95 masks manage to filter at least 95% of the particles suspended in the air.

CHAPTER 8: GUIDELINES FOR WEARING A FACE-COVERING

Improper use of face shields can lead to breathing and the emission of harmful air particles through the mouth and nose. In this way, there is an increase in contracting and spreading the virus to other people.

Your face covering should: tight snugly but comfortably against the side of your face be secured with ties, or ear loops include multiple layers of fabric allow for breathing without restriction be laundered and machine dried without damaging or changing the shape.

Putting on your face covering

Step 1 – Wash your hands with soap and water or an alcohol-based hand sanitizer.

Step 2 – Inspect your face covering for holes or tears.

Step 3 – Place covering over your mouth, like so:

With Ear Loops: Hold by ear loops and place a circle around each ear with Ties:

Bring to your nose, place ties over the crown of your head, and tie.

Step 4 – Pull the covering over the bridge of your nose, mouth.

Making your cloth face mask

You can make your cloth face mask with everyday items around the house and a sewing machine.

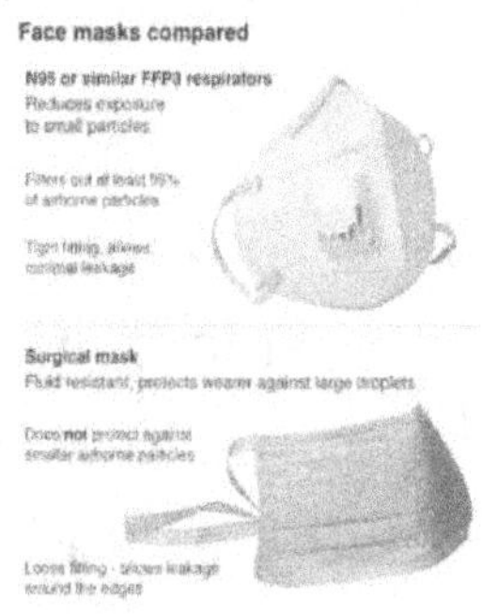

What you'll need:

Two 10" x 6" rectangles of cotton fabric from a t-shirt, scarf, or

Towel Two 6" pieces of elastic or rubber bands, string, cloth strips, or hair ties

Needle and thread, or bobby pin

Scissors

Sewing machine

Steps

1. Stack the two pieces of fabric together and sew them into a single piece of cloth.
2. Fold the long sides ¼ inch and hem.
3. Fold the double layer of material over ½ inch along the short sides and stitch down.
4. To make ear loops, run a six-inch length of elastic through the opening of the broader hem on each side. Use a needle or bobby pin to thread through.
5. Tie the ends tightly.
6. Gently tug the elastic, so the knots are tucked inside the hem.
7. Stitch the elastic in place so, it doesn't slip.

Do I need a filter?

The purpose of a filter is to partially or entirely block the access and exit of potentially infected particles contained in the air coming from and directed towards our respiratory tract. It is possible to increase the altering capacity of a face mask homemade, adding to it an additional layer of propylene, acting as a filter. Propylene is a ubiquitous material in our homes, which can be found in ordinary shopping bags.

The need to add the filter between layers of cotton or other fabric can be seen as an essential precaution to ensure that the beers do not enter our lungs.

Why are face masks necessary?

Facemasks help limit the spread of germs and bacteria. When someone talks, coughs or sneezes, they can release small particles of saliva into the air, that can infect others. An effective face mask can reduce the number of germs released by the wearer, and it can serve to protect others from the risk of being infected when they come into close contact with infected individuals.

How Long Does a Disposable Mask Last?

The type of disposable mask, that built with a strap over the head. This model guarantees very little protection from debris and particles from the atmosphere. These dust masks, as illustrated above in the gore, also take the name of nuisance dust masks and are used in operations such as blowing the leaves to protect themselves from domestic debris. Dust masks just don't offer an excellent face seal and protect well as nose hair, which is to say not that well. It is recommended to replace them when breathing becomes difficult, or after about 8 hours of use and in the presence of exploitation.

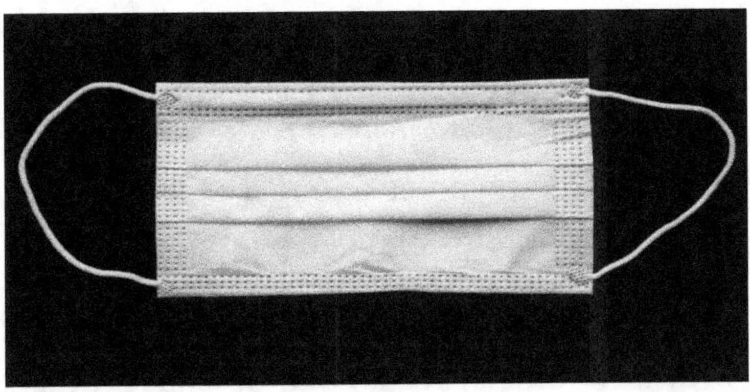

Replace them immediately and often whenever they start to get dirty, damaged, or make breathing difficult, which happens continuously in a construction site where the masks often get dirty the moment you put them down. Molded creates disposable respirators with an exterior lightweight plastic mesh, which helps keep the right filter cloth from contact with dirty surfaces. These masks arrive from the Molded 2200 model that does not always have a breathing valve or the Molded 2300 version, which does possess the exhalation valve. The lid helps maintain the wearer somewhat more relaxed during long periods of working in the mask.

Being able to breathe through a disposable respirator can be very difficult if the filter material becomes clogged or dirty. This is another main reason for improving them. Also, to solve this problem, a practical solution has been devised simply by creating more overlapping surfaces and obtaining more excellent altering. Even the modelled airwave includes an accordion surface that prevents both from getting too dirty and by inserting alter material inside the front area, to guarantee a longer duration, where it takes longer before it is clogged again.

Dust masks and disposable respirators, if damaged and, with torn parts, will have to be changed, as they have a particular purpose to be completed and, if they have perforated sections, they will let in what they should instead alter.

What happens most often is one of the belt breaks. In some cases, it is solvable, while in others, it is to be thrown in the trash and replaced with a new mask.

Another thing to think about is germs. Don't talk about dust masks. Most people do not like to try this anyway. But even when your disposable respirator (or dust mask, also if you are still using one next short article) sounds good after a lot more than just a day, change it out anyway. Many disposable respirators have antimicrobial surfaces, but over the years that they could start to be considered home to germs. Change them out after 8-10 hours, and even if they're, they're not cluttered.

Only recently, the CDC decided to take a drastic stance on the COVID19 pandemic, announcing his concern about the evolution of events, and the fact that it is considered necessary for each person to start wearing face masks in public.

One person who was one of the prominent exponents to have approved the use of the mask immediately is Jeremy Howard, an illustrious researcher at the University of San Francisco. In addition to the profession of skilled and experienced researcher he holds at the University of San Francisco, he is recognized as the founder of fast.ai, a research institute dedicated to making deep learning more accessible. His idea was to have created the Masks4all.co portal, in which he uses and promotes the benefits of everyone in the use of face masks, including those made at home.

CHAPTER 9: HOMEMADE FACE MASK

Surgical masks and respirators of the N95 type are considered to be medical devices, and reserved purely for healthcare and hospital use, for all those who respond in the first person to the need to come into contact with coronavirus patients.

For other people, it is the use of non-medical masks, so even those made at home are more than good.

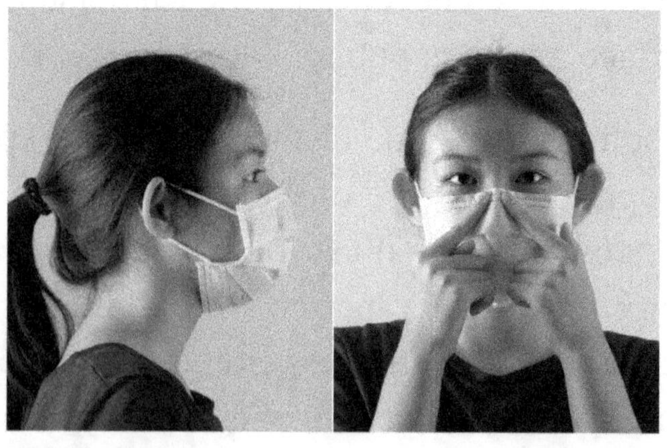

What is really important to know:

Homemade masks are suitable for providing generic protection for yourself, your family, and the people around you, in situations where it is difficult to maintain the task of social distancing, for example, on public transport, in grocery stores, etc.

Given for sure the presence of people with coronavirus, but asymptomatic or who before developing the mild symptoms, still manage to spread the viral infection to others.

For this reason, it should be a good habit that everyone, without exception, uses a face mask.

The homemade masks do not guarantee full safety for the wearer. Still, at least they are better than nothing and manage to protect and prevent only relatively, the risk of spreading and contagion of viral particles.

Everyone must follow the suggestions for using the mask correctly to take advantage of it and safety. These valuable tips recommend:

To improve their hygiene and adopt the good habit of washing their hands before wearing and removing the mask.

Another recommendation to keep in mind is never to

touch or adjust the mask without having adequately cleaned and disinfected your hands.

Don't reusing a cover once you have put it on.

Once used, keep them safe until they can be cleaned with warm, soapy water.

Note: Important thing to know is that non-medical masks alone will not eliminate the risk of spreading COVID-19. Everyone must be aware that they must rigorously adopt adequate hygiene and public health measures so that respectful and responsible behaviour must be maintained, and more outstanding care must be taken for personal hygiene with frequent washing and physical spacing measures to increase the level of safety.

Using Homemade Face Masks Safely

Homemade masks have limitations of use restricted to secure contexts where the risk of contagion is not excessive and to ensure better protection, and they must be safe. For example, those who work in hospitals where the risk of infection is higher will not use DIY masks. You, but the surgical model. Non-medical face masks or facings must be placed on:

Children under the age of two anyone who has

trouble breathing

Anyone who is incapacitated, unconscious, or otherwise unable to remove the mask without appropriate precautions and assistance.

When you choose to use a homemade face mask:

Keep attention to wash your hands immediately before wearing it on and quickly after removing it, and therefore practice good and adequate hand hygiene while wearing it.

Ensure the mask is snug against your face and that it has no damaged parts, such as holes or torn fabrics.

Never share your face mask with other people, because you cannot know if the other person is infected. Furthermore, it is not necessary to wear it and remove it repeatedly during a single use because it increases the risk of accumulation of bacteria and germs onThe masks can be easily contaminated, when they come into contact with the external environment, or when touched by your hands. When wearing a mask,

CHAPTER 10: TAKE THE FOLLOWING PRECAUTIONS TO PROTECT YOURSELF:

When using a mask, you should avoid touching it unless necessary. The moment the cloth mask becomes damp or gets dirty, replace it immediately with a new one, For washing homemade fabric masks, it is recommended to wash them in the washing machine, also together with other objects. Just use washes with hot wash cycles, placing them in a mesh bag to avoid asking during washing at high temperatures, As for the non-medical facial masks that cannot be washed. It is required to replace and dispose of them as soon as they become damp, stained, or crumpled.

How to properly dispose of masks in a lined garbage can:

Don't leave used face masks in shopping carts, on the ground, etc.

They are making Homemade Face Masks Use clean and stretchy 100 per cent cotton t-shirts or pillowcases. Some materials work better than others.

Make sure that the facial mask is perfectly adherent to the face by completely covering the nose and mouth, so as not to allow the passage of infected droplets.

The mask should be comfortable; otherwise, you won't want to wear it consistently.

Tutorial

1. First of all, start to cut out two 10-by-6-inch rectangles of cotton fabric.

Then, use tightly woven cotton, such as quilting fabric or cotton sheets. T-shirt fabric will work in a pinch. Stack the two boxes; you will sew the mask as if it was a single piece of cloth.

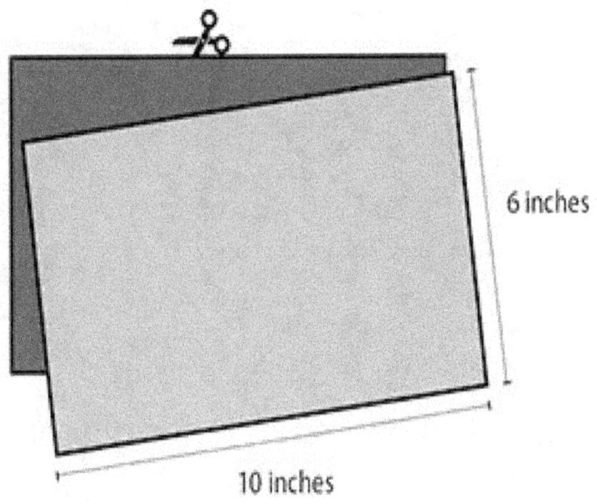

A close up of the two rectangular pieces of cloth needed to make a cloth face covering is shown. These pieces of fabric have been cut using a pair of scissors, each part of cloth measures ten inches in width and six inches in length.

2. Fold over the long sides ¼ inch and hem. Then fold the double layer of fabric over ½ inch along the short sides and stitch down.

. Fold over the long sides ¼ inch and hem. Then fold the double layer of fabric over ½ inch along the short sides and stitch down.

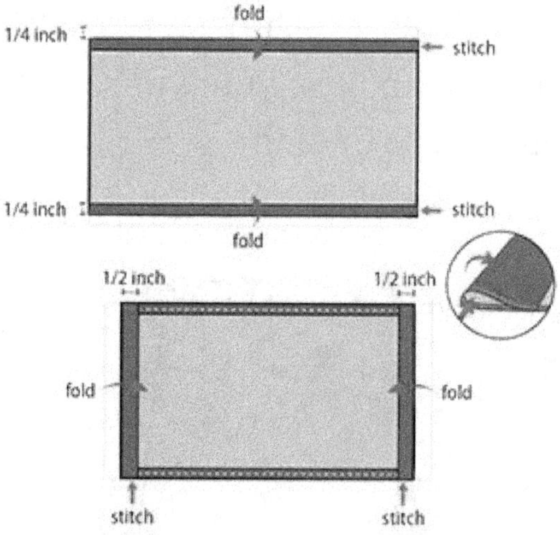

The top diagram shows the two rectangle cloth pieces stacked on top of each other, aligning on all sides. The rectangle, lying at, is positioned so that the two ten-inch sides are the top and the bottom of the box, while the two six-inch sides are the left and right side of the rectangle. The top diagram shows the two long edges of the cloth rectangle are folded over and stitched into place to

create a one-fourth inch hem along the entire width of the top and bottom of the square. The bottom diagram shows the two short edges of the cloth rectangle are folded over and stitched into place to create a one-half inch hem along the entire length of the right and left sides of the face covering.

3.   Run a 6-inch length of 1/8-inch wide elastic through the full hem on each side of the mask. These will be the ear loops. Use a large needle or a bobby pin to thread it through. Tie the ends tight.

Don'tDon't have elastic? Use hair ties or flexible headbands. If you only have a string, you can make the relationship longer and tie the mask behind your head.

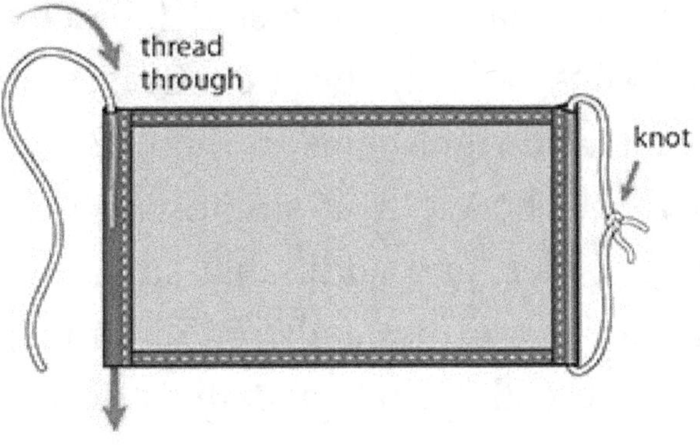

Two six-inch pieces of elastic or string are threaded through the open one-half inch hems created on the left and right side of the rectangle. Then, the two ends of the flexible or rope are tied together into a knot.

4. Gently pull on the elastic so that the knots are tucked inside the hem. Gather the sides of the mask on the flexible and adjust, so the cover it'sits your face.

Then securely stitch the elastic in place to keep it from slipping.

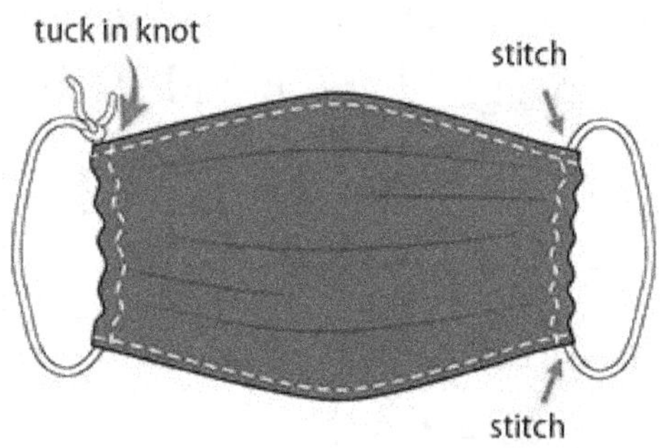

The diagram displays a completed face covering, in which the knots of the elastic strings are tucked inside the left and right hems of the mask and are no longer visible. The cloth is slightly gathered on its left and right sides, and additional stitching is added to the four corners of the gathered cloth rectangle, at the points where the cloth and the elastic or string overlap in these corners.

Materials

- T-shirt Scissors
- Tutorial

A front view of a T-shirt is shown. A straight, horizontal line is cut across the entire width of the T-shirt, parallel to the T-shirt'sT-shirt's waistline. Using scissors, the cut is made approximately seven to eight inches above the waistline, the front and back layer of the T-shirt is cut simultaneously.

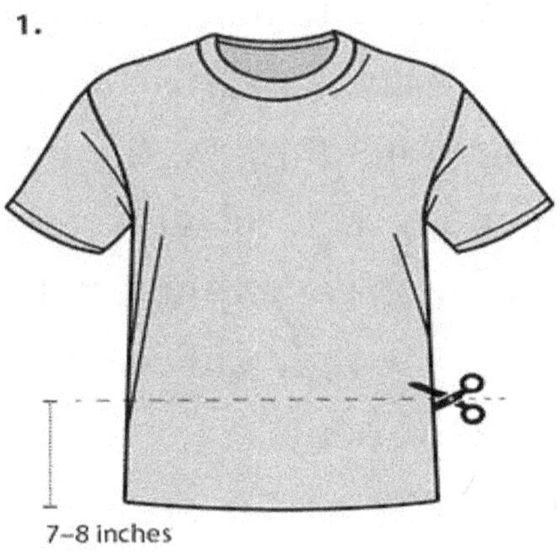

The rectangle piece of cloth that has been cut from the bottom portion of the T-shirt is shown, lying at. The rectangle is positioned so that the cut that was just made across the entire width of the shirt is the top side of the box, while the original waistline of the T-shirt is the bottom side of the rectangle. From the top right-hand corner of the square, the scissors are moved down an approximately one-half inch, along the right, hemmed side of the box. From this point, a six to seven-inch, a horizontal cut is made through both the front and backside of the cloth, parallel to the top of the rectangle. The scissors then turn ninety-degrees to cut downward, a vertical line that is parallel to the left side of the box; this cut continues downward until it reaches approximately one-half inch above the bottom of the rectangle. The scissors then turn ninety degrees again to create another six to seven-inch, horizontal cut that runs parallel to the bottom of the box, back towards the right hemmed side of the shirt and cuts through the power hemmed side of the rectangle. This newly cut out piece of cloth is laid to the side. To cut the tie strings, the two remaining slivers of the right side of the rectangle are cut vertically along the hem.

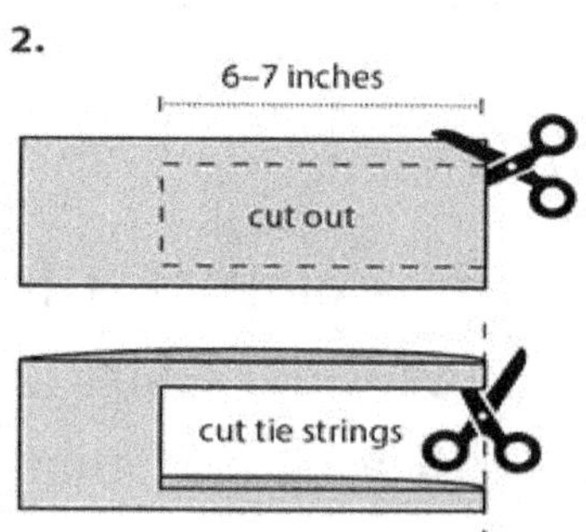

The piece of cloth is unfolded and worn by an individual. The middle of the cloth piece is positioned to cover the nose and mouth area; the four thin slices of cloth act as tie strings to hold the cloth face-covering in place. The ropes around the neck, then over the top of the head, are tied into knots.

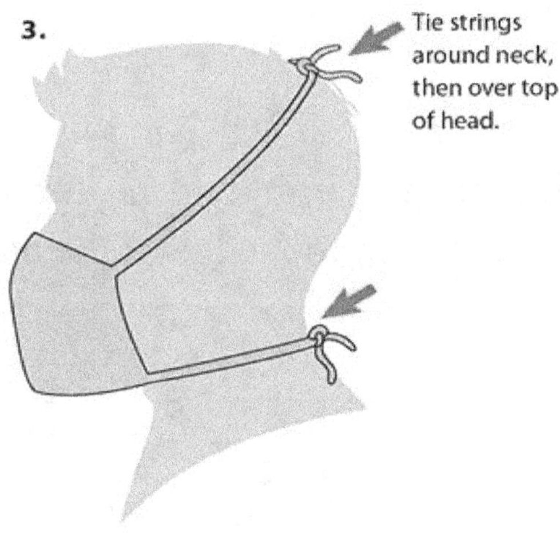

Materials

- Bandana (or square cotton cloth approximately 20" x20")
- Rubber bands (or hair ties)
- Scissors (if you are cutting your fabric)
- Tutorial

  A single bandana is shown lying at, with the curved edge at the top. Cut banana in half with a horizontal line.

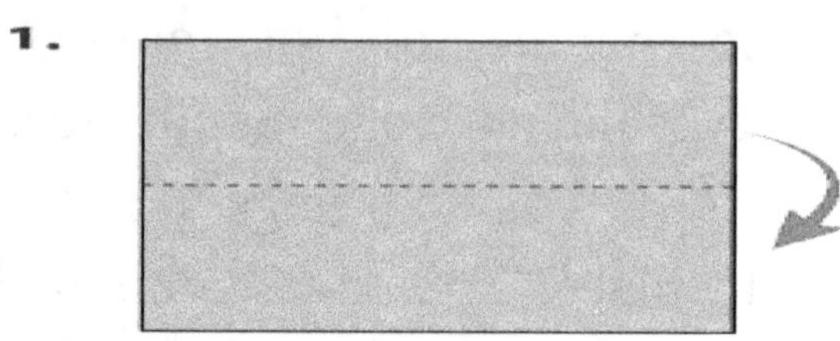

Fold bandana in half.

The square bandana is shown lying at. The bandana is then folded in half, bringing the top edge of the bandana to meet the bottom edge of the bandana.

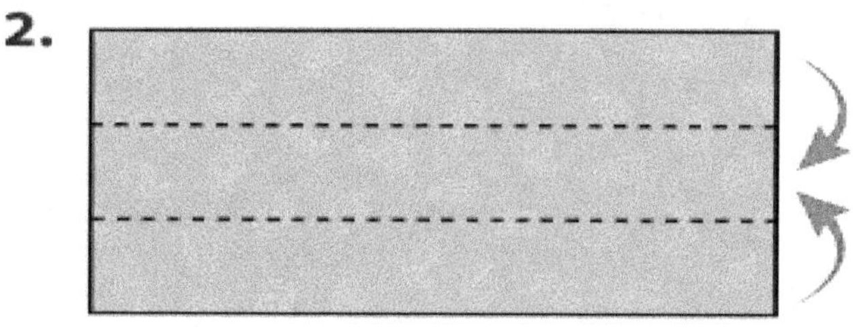

Fold top down. Fold bottom up.

The top half of the bandana, with the curved edg

e at the top, is placed in the centre of the folded bandana. Then, fold filter in the centre of the folded bandana. Fold top down. Fold the bottom up to cover the screen entirely.

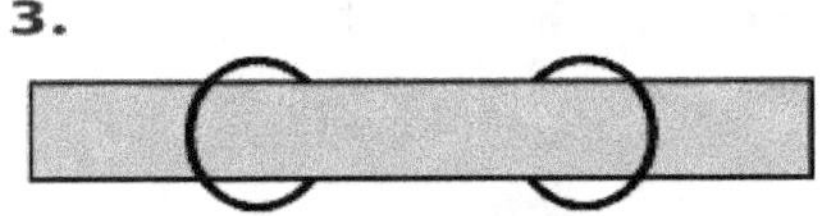

Insert the folded bandana, with the filter inside, through the centre of two rubber bands or hair ties. Place rubber bands or hair ties about 6 inches apart.

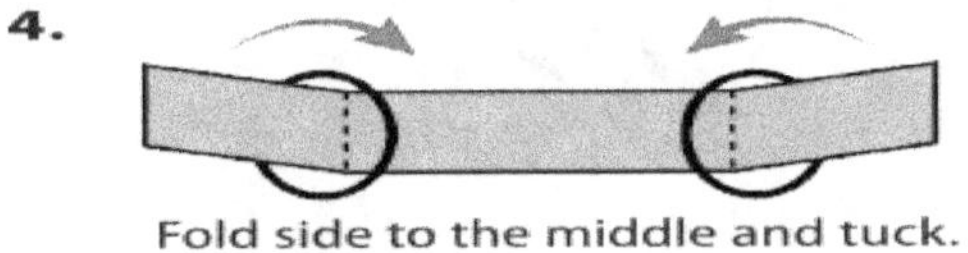

Take the left side and the right side of the bandana

and fold each party to the middle and tuck the sides into each other.

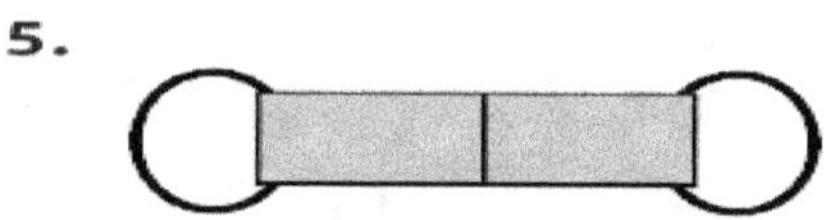

5.

The bandana should now be a continuous, cloth loop since the left and right sides have been tucked into each other.

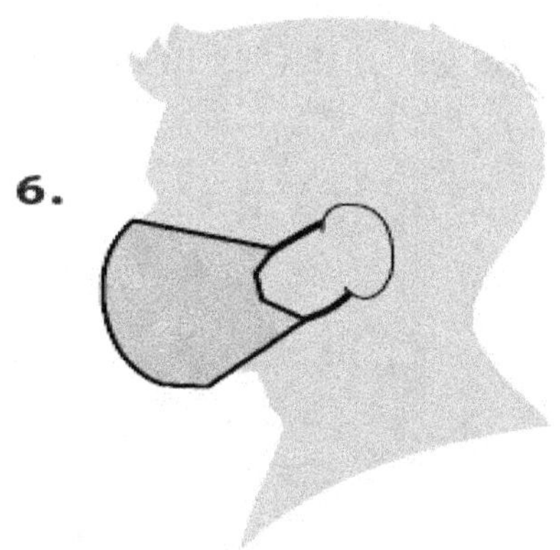

6.

CONCLUSION

This book is all about the type of generally made mask, and use is likely to decrease viral exposure and infection risk on a population level, despite poor and imperfect adherence, personal respirators providing most protection. Masks worn by patients may not offer as high a degree of protection against aerosol transmission.

DIY REUSABLE FACE MASK PATTERN

INTRODUCTION

This project base on how to use and not to use a medical face mask. It we give more information base on the way to protect us from the virus and bridge the gap between human being and infection in the world.

The development of this face mask is to prevent or protect the human being from virus, and to overcome the challenges against this crisis, which have affected the standard of living and the world economy at large, and have impacted negatively.

CHAPTER 1: BEST FACE MASK FOR VIRUS PROTECTION

1. Mask respirator

First, this face mask 3M / N95 respirator certified by NIOSH (National Institute for Occupational Safety and Health). This means that it can effectively maintain particles larger than 0.3 microns. This is sufficient to block the water droplets carrying the virus.

I am pleased that this respirator/mask comes with a patented valve Cool Flow 3M. This helps to let out the heat and steam of my breath. He even helped keep the interior cool, dry mask. This infected mask also comes with a nose clip adjustable metal. This feature makes it easy to create a good seal around the face.

There are no loopholes that allow foreign particles to enter the inside of the nose and mouth. Braided elastic band provides sufficient rigidity to maintain the insured mask against my face. Fortunately, it's not so much that the cover will leave a mark on my skin when it comes out.

The problem I think most people, or at least

most people have with this mask is that the elastic bands are tight. Fortunately, this is not so much that it becomes uncomfortable, but this oppression can sometimes be annoying.

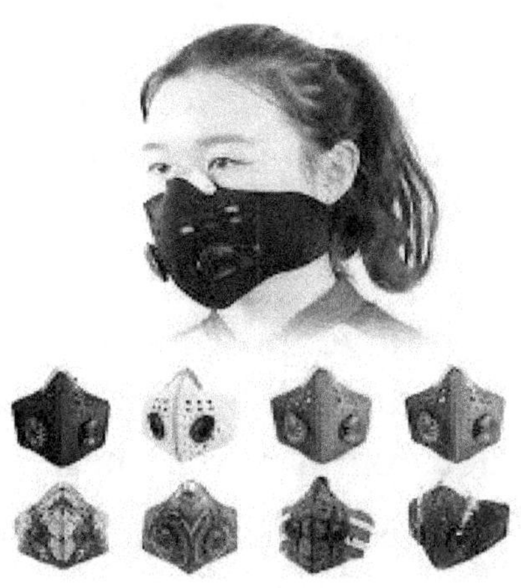

2. Face Masks disposable Co-power

Many people say that medical masks are not effective in protecting against viruses. However, putting two layers of tissue paper inside, this disposable mask may be helpful. One thing I liked about this the cover is that it is very cheap. For its reasonable price, you can get 100 pieces of throwaway masks.

Meanwhile, this mask can block particles that are greater than 2.5 microns wide. To give some perspective on how small it is, a human hair is 70 microns thick. Another thing to know about this mask is soft and comfortable it is to use. It is made of three layouts of non-woven material serving as the filter.

They are also soft to the touch. I can wear them without feeling any discomfort at all. I am also satisfied mainly because it comes with a metal clip on the soft nose. Simply clicking on the nose clip metal, you can create a good seal around the mouth and nose.

What little I have problems with is that this need not block the virus. If a person with the illness sneezes in the face, or at least, there is still a good chance of infection within three feet.

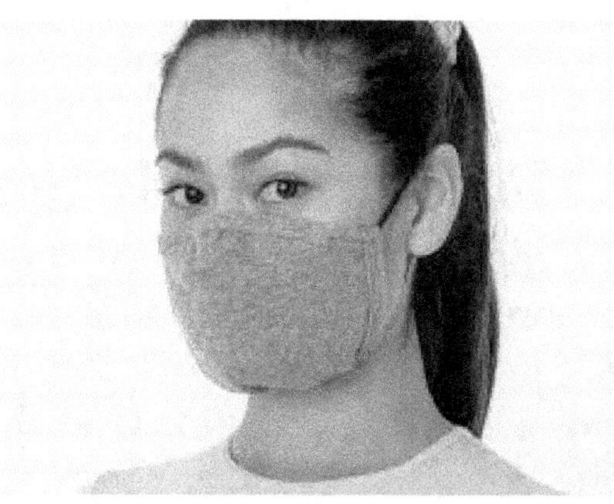

3. Nuisance dust mask Honeywell, disposable

NIOSH cannot approve this dust mask, so it has no rating, but they do an excellent job of filtering particles in the standard air. Although there is nothing that states if this is good to keep out illness, it is still managing than using nothing at all.

I like that the material is very soft. This allows it to fit comfortably against my face. They have no problem following the contours of the face. This mask also has a metal strip on the bridge of the nose.
You can tweak so you can clip onto your nose and create a good seal around the nose and mouth. fAt the beginning, I thought the single elastic band would not be enough to keep the cover in place, but when I tried it on, surprisingly clung quite well.

The biggest problem I have with this mask is that NIOSH does not approve cit, although it does a great job of blocking dust and odors certain chemicals, no way to know if it is effective against the virus.

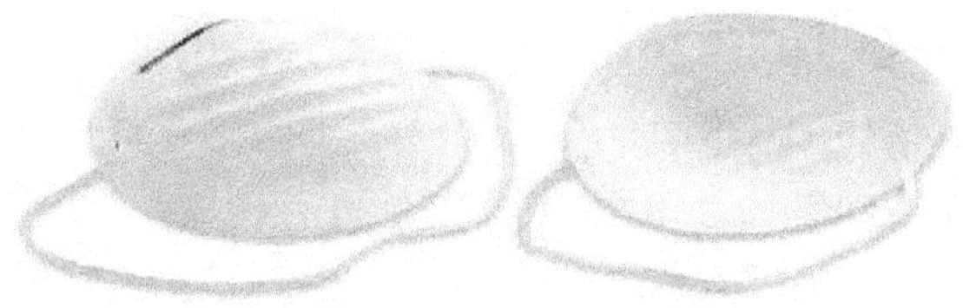

4. Medical Mask 3M N95 1860

Apart from being certified by NIOSH, this surgical mask is also approved by the FDA as safe for medical use. These are classified as N95 to be filtered at the least 95% of all particles in the air, including most bacteria and viruses.

The little thing I like about this mask is that there is some foam padding on the metal nose clip. This provides some comfort and makes it bearable to wear the mask for hours.

The two elastic that goes over the head provide the right amount of elasticity to keep the mask firmly in place. Having two bands also helps distribute pressure evenly over the cover. This prevents twisting out of place after a while.

I am speaking of headbands, which are quite durable. I've been wearing these masks until the recommended time, and elastic bands do not loosen. What I do not like about this mask is that it has an exhalation valve. After a time, the heat that builds up inside the cover is placed a little too unbearable.

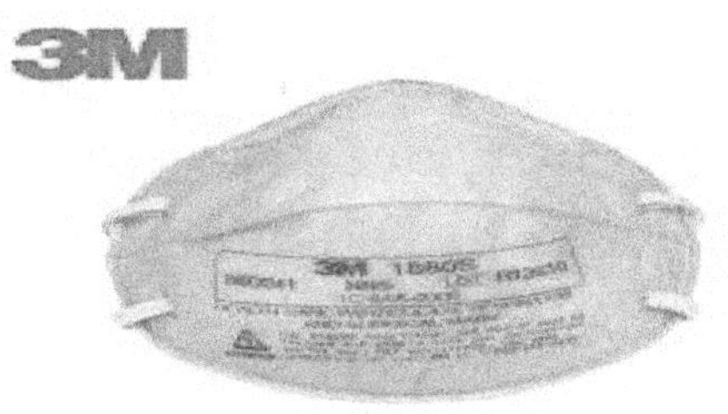

5. Disposable mask 3layer breathable safety filter

In the beginning, I was worried because these are simply generic surgical masks but perform very well. With some adjustment, these masks are capable of blocking foreign particles from reaching the nose and mouth.

The setting of this mask is also high. This is designed for an average adult face, and rubber bands are sufficiently flexible that they can even fit appropriately in young children. Moreover, if these are generic masks made in the US, He gave me some relief.

It pays to be selective with the spread of the virus as fast as it is right now. Moreover, even with all the panic going around, this mask is still being sold at a reasonable price while still having enough decent quality. The price is affordable and cheap for a day or two of breathing protection.

The only thing I do not like is that these are not

branded. I have no qualms about using unbranded products, but they must have at least the name of the industrial on them to get attention to the customer later.

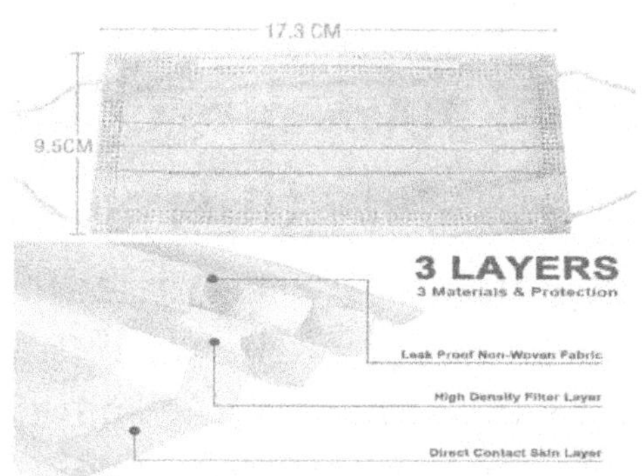

6. Dynarex 2201 Medical-surgical face mask

These masks are not classified N95, but they will do in a pinch. Many people say that these types of covers are ineffective, but in the absence of accurate particle filter masks, you can still be a great substitute.

Another reason I like this product is that it is very economical. You can get a modest amount of safeguards every day for just a low price, which is more practical than sick.

Although this product is affordable, note that this does not mean that loosens give adequate protection. This is made of medical-grade textile and can block more matter particles in the air.

The elastic bands also provide sufficient tension to hold the mask tightly pressed against the face without restricting breathing. The groups are also durable that could last a whole day.
I just have a problem with a face mask - and that's it's a little too thin compared with similar products. Yes, it is quite possible that still can block particulate matter, but it is not so reassuring.

Although this is not an N95 respirator, if you are anxious about the virus, this will do fine in a pinch. You can do this merely sufficient by adding a couple of sheets of tissue paper. This will be infinitely better than not using any mask at all.

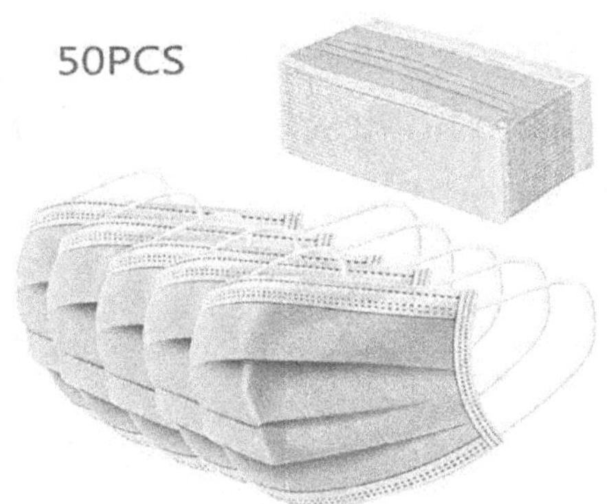

7. Folding mask respirator SolidWorks

I'm so impressed with this mask is having an exhalation valve. This helped keep the inside cool, dry cover, which is an issue that usually has simple surgical.

If you are doubtful, then I can assure you that this mask is NIOSH approved as an N95 respirator. This means that it can be locked at the least 95% of all particles, not based oil known suspension.

This also has a double layer of filter material durable for optimum protection and durability. This product was initially destined as a dust mask used by craftsmen, so they need to be sustainable.
One thing about this mask is that it is very comfortable. Although it might seem rigid and hard, it adapts to the contours of the face and creates a seal around the nose and mouth.

The only problem I have with this product is that it is not on the list of approved N95 filtering masks CDC. This is not personally a big problem as many brands were not tested by the CDC but would have been better if this product was approved.

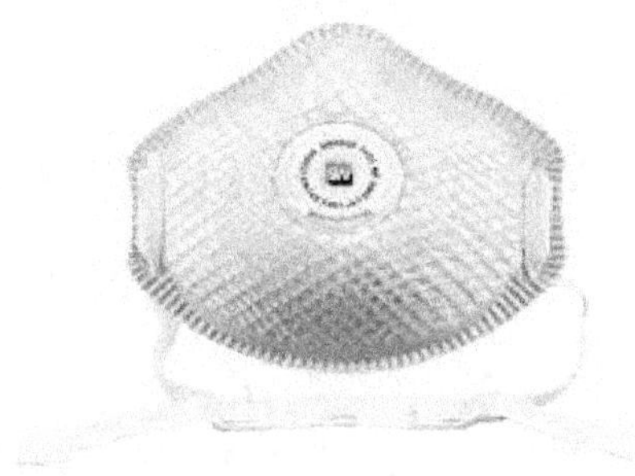

8. Kimberly-Clark mask Fluid Shield Procedure Face

The best of this medical mask is that it has the highest rating fluid resistance, which is level 3, as maintained by the American Society for Materials (ASTM).
I am delighted with this product because it came from one of the most reliable pharmaceutical companies worldwide, Kimberly-Clark. They will not risk putting their mark on any surgical mask.

A small detail that many might have overlooked is the small foam strip is placed in the metal nose clip. This small piece of foam provides a little padding that makes the mask a little more comfortable.
Another thing I liked is that this mask is soft and breathable. One would think that with the level of protection provided, the user would have to give up comfort, but it does at all.

The problem I have with these masks is not active. They work well. It's just that I realized they are so thin that it is difficult to convince myself of the product's efficacy.

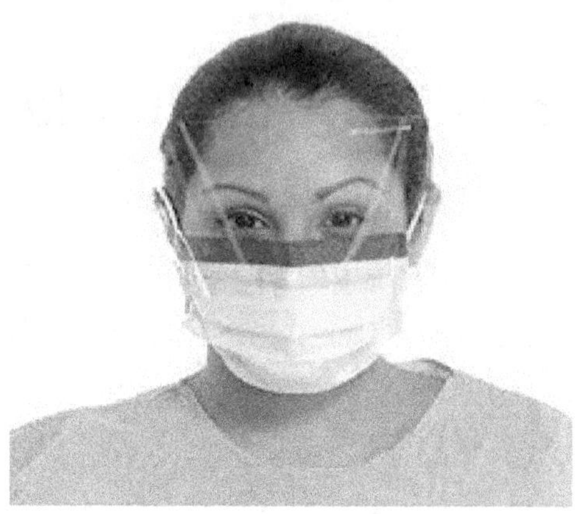

9. 4530 universal heavy-duty non-toxic safety masks

This mask is perfect for creating a good seal around the mouth and nose. In the beginning, I thought this is too hard, but when I gave one a try, I was surprised that it conformed to the shape of the face quite well.

I was also surprised at how light this mask is. After an hour or, I completely forgot that I was using it. The cover has a metal band placed around the nose. When pressed against the nose, the group will bend and form around the bridge of the nose, creating a good seal around them at all.

The issue I have with these masks is not valid. They band, but strong and elastic. The group has sufficient elasticity to keep the flat mask against his face securely, but not so tight that it is uncomfortable. There is a problem with these masks. N95 masks are not NIOSH approved. This could discourage some of these respirators, even giving it a chance.

Although this mask is NIOSH approved, if you are in a bind, it will work better than just using a tissue to cover your mouth. Also, these masks N95 could be equivalent (at the least in my experience, they seem to be).

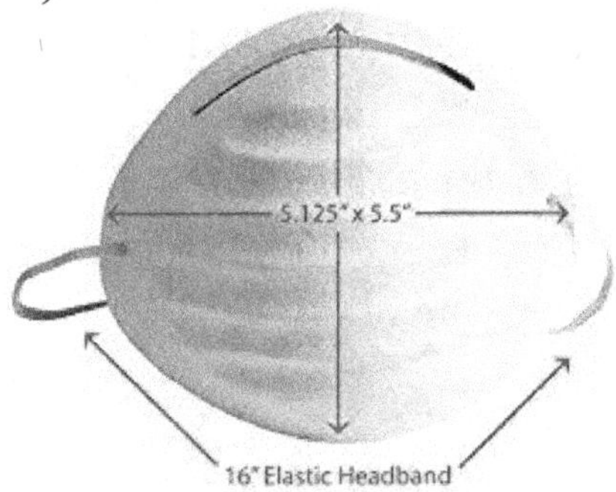

10. Ellipse GVS SPR451 P100 Half respiratory mask

The best feature is that this respirator is NIOSH approved and classification of P100. This means that it can filter nearly 100% of all particles suspended in air, including chemicals-based oil.

The N95 respirator is 100% silicone, which means it is completely hypoallergenic and adorable. You can make a complete seal around the nose and mouth. Nothing can get inside the mask.

They were speaking of the filters if it is not used for construction purposes, which It can be used for a week to a month. Simply replace the cleaners when they get too clogged with dust.

The mask also has an exhalation valve pointing downwards. What those means is that you are wearing glasses that do not fog whenever you breathe out. This also keeps the interior dry and cool mask.

Protective masks are essential when it is likely that work carried out to discard the dust, vapors, gases, and other toxic products ... To protect adequately, models can use a single-use disposable or reusable models adapted to each situation. You still have to know how to recognize them, choose them, and use them!

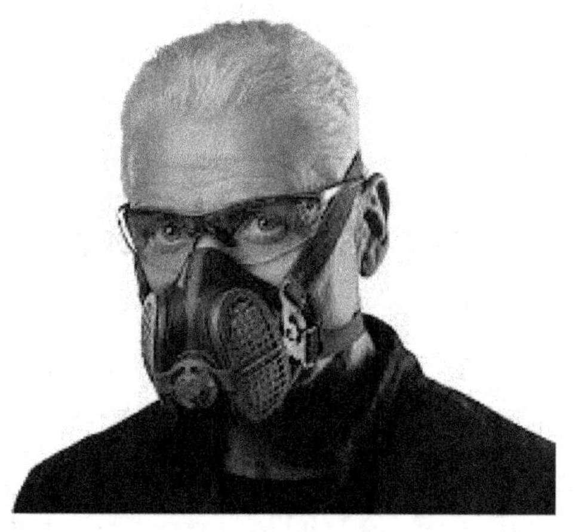

CHAPTER 2: EXAMPLE OF FACE MASK PATTERN

Several easy-to-make options exist to cover your face with your creation. These alternatives will allow the masks of procedures and the famous N95 to be left to health professionals who are at higher risk.

Seamless

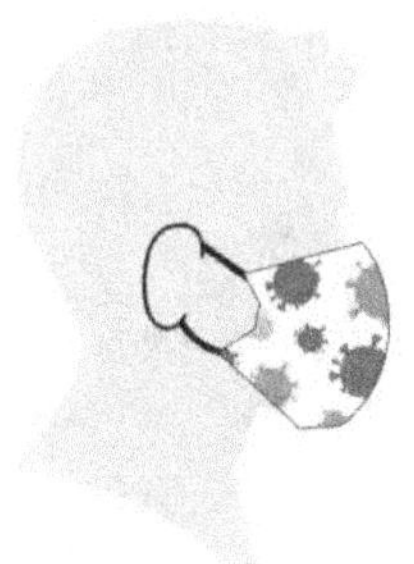

Even if you don't know how to sew, you can still make masks at home. They may be less comfortable and aesthetic than those with seams, but they are always convenient.

The easiest way is to fold a square piece of fabric and slip rubber bands at the ends of the rectangle you will get, If you have a t-shirt that you no longer wear, you can cut out a mask that you will attach behind your head.

Material required for the first method

- Fabric square
- Hair elastic, elastic cords or rubber elastic

Material required for the second method

- An old t-shirt
- A good pair of scissors

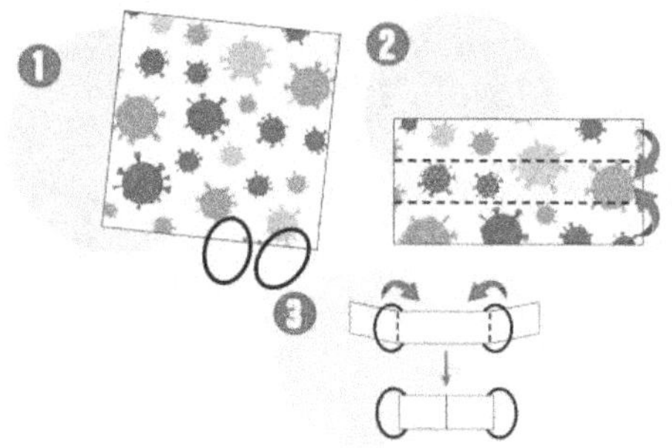

Steps

1. Start with a piece of fabric and two hair ties.
2. Place a paper towel in the center of the material then fold the top and bottom of the fabric over the paper towel.
3. After sliding the elastic bands, wrap the sides of the fabric towards the center by inserting one hand into the other before placing it on your face.

Sewn masks

Do you own a sewing machine, or do you know how to use a needle? You can start designing a sewn mask. Several patterns and tutorials that vary in difficulty are available, including this one. Besides, it is not forbidden to let your creativity go by changing the fabrics.

The simplest and most effective option is a rectangular mask with folds to better cover the nose and chin. If you do not want to sew, it is still possible to use fabric glue or diaper pins to hold everything in place; however, this could affect comfort.

Material required:

- Fabric, preferably cotton
- A sewing machine or needle and thread
- Scissors
- Elastic cords or fabric straps
- It is also possible to obtain kits, including all the necessary material on the web. The company Club Tissus sells sets allowing the production of five masks. For each sale, $ 3 will be donated to the Chaînon, an

accommodation resource for women in difficulty in Quebec.

Disposables

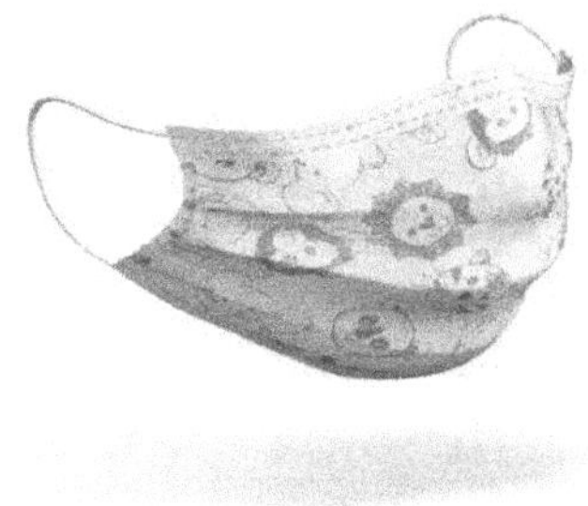

Disposable masks, although less ecological, do not need to be maintained, unlike those made of fabric. Note, however, that health authorities do not recommend them. Researcher Geneviève Marchand of the Robert-Sauvé Institute also raises a caveat about very absorbent materials that can release the liquid after a certain period.

The method for making them resemble those of fabric. First, superimpose two sheets of absorbent paper which you will fold into an accordion.

Place rubber bands at the ends and fold them back on themselves. Hold everything with staples or sticky paper.

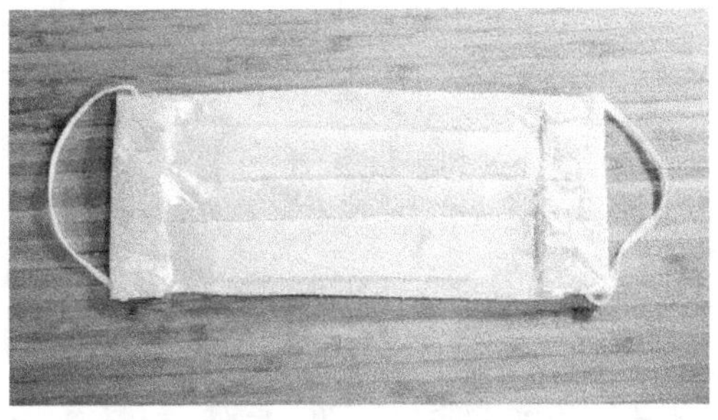

You can add a coffee filter to the side that will touch your face by holding it in place with staples.

Material required

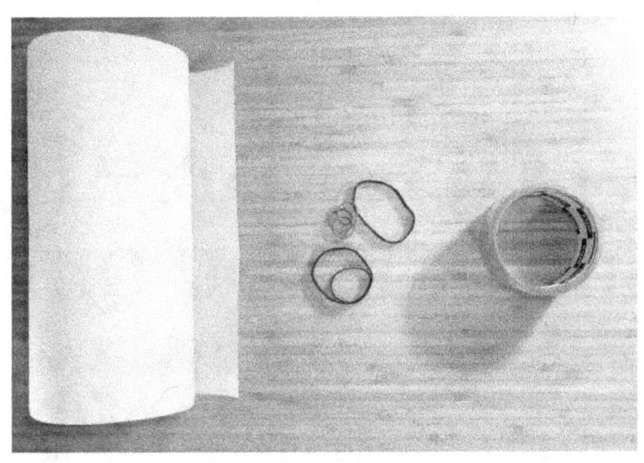

> ➤ Absorbent paper
> ➤ Coffee filter
> ➤ Stapler
> ➤ Rubber elastic

Fabrics to cover the face

If you do not want to tinker, it is possible to wear a scarf, a neck warmer, or a bandana to cover the face. However, these accessories are more likely to slip and may need to be replaced, which will result in hand-to-face contact.

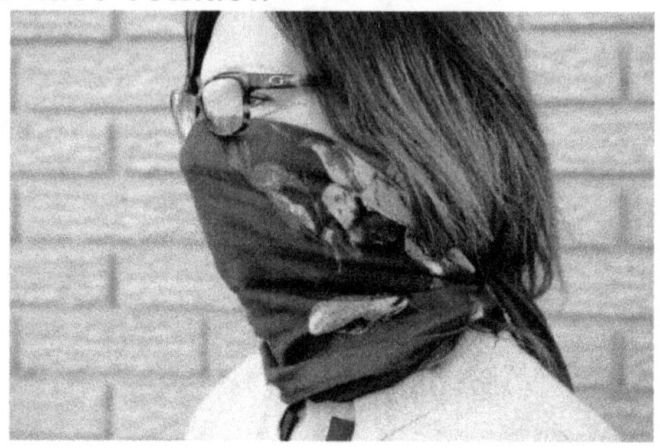

CHAPTER 3: SOME ADVICE BEFORE YOU GET STARTED

The public health maintenance of Canada has some recommendations for the design of non-medical masks. They must:

> Be made up of at least two layers of fabric (such as cotton or linen)
> Cover mouth and nose entirely without leaving holes
> Be securely attached to the head by ties or cords forming loops that go behind the ears.
> Allow easy breathing
> Be comfortable and wear without requiring frequent adjustments.

> Be changed as soon as possible if they become wet or dirty.
> Keep their shape after being washed and dried.

DIY facial masks are not as effective as surgical masks authentic.

Is there a need for cloth face masks?

Currently, the supply of surgical masks is the lowest of all critical times nationwide.

Orders for standard disposable masks used in hospitals are ordered around, and there is a great demand for protective equipment for health workers.

According to the CDC, cloth masks are an option for responding to crises when they have exhausted other supplies.

Because of these concerns, many hospitals across the country have requested surgical masks made at home as a temporary emergency measure.

The CDC now recommends using face cloth coatings.

Also, federal health officials now recommend that people's mouth and nose with cloth masks are covered in public.

This is a voluntary public health measure to curb the spread of help when people need to visit public places such as grocery stores and public transport stations.

CDC also advises using pure fabric coatings to reduce the spread of the virus and help people who may have the illness and do not know to transmit it to others.
Sewing a fabric mask to be allowed medical surgical masks and N95 masks degree are professionals and patients' health care reserved.

An important distinction

homemade masks are not as effective as an N95 filter mask
Instead, they are intended:
To meet the demands of covers in emergency hospitals.
Community members help "curb the spread" in public places where other social distancing measures are challenging to maintain.
Sources Readings: Cambridge study, Nature, occ. Approx. Med, Annals Occ Health)

Face masks are home the Last haunt
The Centers for Virus Control and Prevention (CDC) said that in times of crisis, homemade masks are acceptable as a last resort. On the CDC website, strategies to optimize the supply of face masks explain that if homemade face masks are not a substitute for the PPE, it can be used in situations

where facemasks are unavailable.

HCP use homemade masks:

In places where facemasks are unavailable, HCP can use homemade masks (e.g., bandana scarf) to treat patients with Covid-19 as a last resort. However, homemade masks are not considered PPE. For their protection capacity, HCP is unknown. One must be careful to find this option. Homemade masks should ideally fabric be used in combination with a mask that covers the entire front (which extends to the chin or below) and the side of the face.

I put in strong guard before spending time sewing masks:

Follow CDC guidelines as the situation evolves.
Contact your local clinic and hospital to ensure they accept masks, masks, and all that you will meet their guidelines.

Some hospitals require surgical masks homemade.

Some hospitals and clinics that accept donations of homemade masks. Organizations such as masks for Heroes now have a facility database in search of gifts. If you are wondering where you can mask help, a hospital or clinic needs to donate found, to make a big batch of masks sewing donations before spending time, please ask first if they accept.

You should ask if this model (2 layers of fabric with a pocket for additional disposable inserts) will meet their needs. You should also ask about the procedures of landing/pickup.

CHAPTER 4: THE BEST MATERIALS TO MAKE A FACE MASK

scientist at Cambridge University has tested the usefulness of a wide range of household materials in homemade costumes. They measured how domestic materials could capture and filter small particles.

The test data shows that the best choice for DIY fabric masks is cotton T-shirts, pillowcases, cotton, or other materials. Using a double layer of content for your DIY mask adds a small increase in filtration efficiency.

Other research has found that the most effective two layers masks heavyweight "quilters cotton" thread density at least 180 were constructed, and it was one more tight thicker tissue.
This pattern has two layers of fabric and an inner bag

in which one can add layers of disposable filter material if desired.

materials for a fabric hospital mask
The DIY surgic

pins or clips al mask pattern

- ➢ The finished mask adult is 7.75 "wide and 3.75" tall.
- ➢ materials
- ➢ 100% cotton fabric (with a tight weave)
- ➢ 1/8 "flat elastic loops for ear loops, or four fabric (can use the same woven fabric to strips, using pre-made bias or strips cotton knit)
- ➢ fabric scissors

sewing machine and thread

Cut List

- For a mask adult size:
- Cut one material rectangle 16 "long and 8.5" wide
- Cut two pieces of elastic, each 7 "long (or even 8" for adult size)
- For a small child-sized mask:
- Cut one fabric rectangle 14 "long and 6.5" wide

- Cut two pieces of elastic, each 6 "long

For a large infant size mask:

- Cut one rectangle fabric 15 "long and 7.5" wide
- Cut two pieces of elastic each 6/5 "long

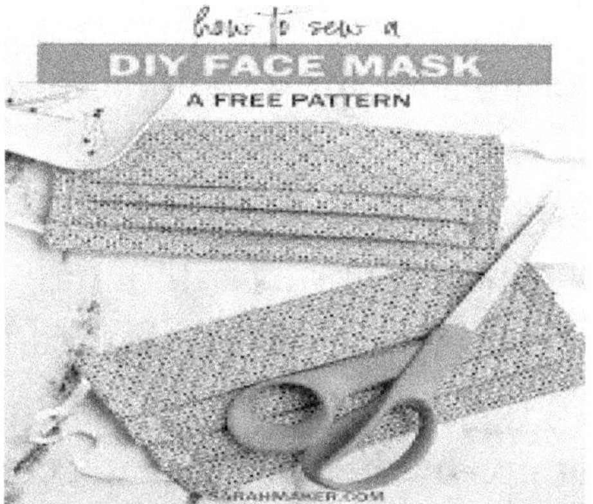

For fabric loops, if you are not using elastic:

Cut four rectangles 18 "long by 1.75" wide. Fold long sides to meet in the middle and fold in half again to enclose the raw edges cosa down the length of the rectangles along the edge to create the loops.
18 "for some people may be too long, especially children.
diagram showing how to sew cloth masks for hospitals

Step 1: Sew on the upper side, with pocket.
Fold the cloth rectangle in half, with the right side against the other.
Sew along the top 8.5 "wide edge, using a large 5/8" seam allowance. Leave a hole 3 "-4" in the center of this seam to create an opening for the pocket filter, and to allow the mask is right side out after sewing. In the image above, I have marked this opening pins.

Update: Some people find it easier to insert/remove the additional filter if they make a larger opening. Instead of a 3-inch opening left "opening, you could make a 4".

materials and supplies to sew a surgical mask

I do not want a pocket filter? If you do not want or need a pocket, that's fine. Anyway, you will have to leave an opening so you can rotate the mask right out. After connecting the elastic or ties (in the next step) and the right cover turned out, you can see the closed opening. Then you can continue with the rest of the directions, sewing seam meter fabric filter surgical mask then turn the fabric so that the seam of the opening of the pocket is centered in the middle of one side. Using an iron, press the seam open.

Fold the excess margin seam under which encloses the edge of the fabric weave. Topstitch or zigzag along each side of the seam to finish the edge. This will help keep the fabric fraying to the insert and remove any filter.

Step 2: Elastic Pin or gender Ties If used elastic:

Pin a piece of elastic to each side of the mask, one end to the top corner and one end to the bottom edge of the rectangle of the fabric. This will create the ear hook once the cover is on the right side out and pleating. Placing the ends of the elastic about 1/4 "to 1/2" from the top and bottom corners of the fabric.

The elastic piece itself is sandwiched between two layers of fabric. Once you turn on the right side of the mask, the elastic is abroad.

Repeat to make this process on each side two loops ear.

Using tissue fasteners - Alternative:

If you cannot find elastic or prefer using fabric links, you can use four fasteners fabric, one in each corner. Each tie is 18 "long. Sew one lace in each turn, being careful not to catch the links in the side seams.

You can also use the twill tape, bias tape, or strips of cotton jersey (shirt fabric).

The finished mask will then be carried by attaching the fabric that remains behind the head. See notes at the end of the post.

Step 3: sewing the sides, fixing links with a seam allowance 3/8 ", sew each side of the face mask. Backstitch on the elastic ties or fabric to secure them. Cut corners with scissors so that it will be easier to turn the cover on the right side Be care not to clip the stitches coincidentally.
Turn the mask right side out and press with an iron. You can use a pencil to push the corners using a wire to create a flexible nosepiece to a fabric mask

Optional: Insert an adjustable nose piece Cut a 6-inch piece of pipe cleaner, floral wire, or other flexible wire to create a nose piece. I folded the rear ends of the son in to prevent them from poking through the fabric. Place the wire through the hole pocket and slide it to the top of the mask. Assembly around on three sides to hold it in place.

Step 4: Folds Make the mask with three evenly spaced lines. To do this, you can measure and mark with a fabric pen water-soluble. Or, you can do what I did, and bend the mask quarters - fold the sides to meet in the middle and again fold in half. Use an iron to make a crease, use pins to secure three plies on a surgical mask fabric.

Use your brand to create three evenly spaced 1/2 "folds. Pin the folds down, make sure that all folds are in the same direction. Sew along the sides to fix the creases. I love to sew the sides twice, just to be sure.

When the mask is worn, pleats are open downwardly to prevent the collection of particles in the folding pockets sewing folds down onto the side of a surgical tissue mask for hospitals Troubleshooting pattern

And if you cannot find elastic?

I heard many people who are struggling to find elastic. If you cannot find flexible to earrings, you can make a mask with fabric fasteners instead. You can use ready-made 1/4 "twill tape, double-fold bias tape, or cut long strips of fabric of cotton tightly woven that you use for the rest of the mask.

For links through fabric: Cut 18 "long strips of cloth, 1.75" wide. Fold long sides together (the length of the hot dog style), so they meet in the middle. They were then folding the strips to one and one-half (range) to wrap the raw edges. Point down the pieces along the side to create links.

how to make strips of bias binding tissue

If you want these straps for a bit of stretch, you can cut long pieces of cotton jersey or knitted material t-shirt. The great thing about using jersey fabric is that it forms a tube when you stretch. And, it is comfortable to wear, as it keeps a little stretch.

Whichever option you choose, you'll want to cut four pieces approximately 18 "long and tie a band at each corner. The mask secures by attaching the straps behind the head.

What metal to help the adjustment to better mask?

To help the mask fit better around your nose, you can insert a length of flexible metal inside the top of the cover, through the insert pocket opening before forming the folds. Then you can topstitch down around the metal insert to keep it in place. I have seen people use pipe cleaners, floral wire, or fasteners.

What can be used as a filter?

It is so important that everyone understands that while using a cloth mask can provide some level of protection, cannot protect against viruses in the same way an N95 mask can.

Many different types of filters have been suggested, such as coffee filters, felt, and vacuum filter bags. Not all of these filters are effective, and not all of them are safe.

Without further research on the safety and effectiveness of materials filter face mask, we will not know what

It is the best filter.

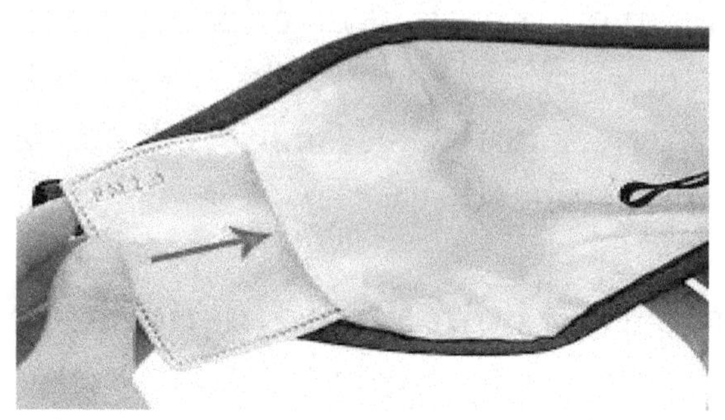

Facial mask filter materials: pros and cons

HEPA filters. In tests, a layer of HEPA vacuum cleaner bag seemed to perform the best. However, it is difficult to breathe. Many people have expressed concern about the safety of materials (such as fiberglass) used to produce these filters. Right now, I cannot recommend it.

Coffee filters. One of the designs masks the CDC has published a layer of a coffee filter. They are readily available and disposable.

Blue shop towels. Others have tested the effectiveness of blue sheets workshops like this. They are promising, but the data have not been released publicly or verified.

Dryer sheet or baby wipes. Because these elements are covered with fragrances and other chemicals not recommend the use of these as a filter.

Non-woven interface.

Flannel or felt. These materials are not as tightly woven cotton fabric as outside the mask, so it is doubtful that improve efficiency filtration. Also, it can trap moisture.

A layer of cotton fabric. We research suggests that a more secure and more straightforward option for a filter material is a cotton shirt or cotton cloth tightly woven, If you are sewing for hospitals that may have their medical-grade filters, always call before sewing to check your requirements.
Disclaimer: This pattern has not been tested in the industry and is intended for educational purposes only. The decision to use this device is the only of its own.

Where can you donate masks?

Not all hospitals are requesting masks, but many are. Find your local hospital to see if they have asked for donations.
Many groups, such as sewing and craft Alliance, are working to connect volunteer sawists health organizations and registering.
Also, an organization called Masks for Heroes has a website with a database of facilities currently looking for donations. If you are wondering where you can donate masks, which can help find a hospital or clinic that needs them.

CHAPTER 5: HOW IS A CLOTH MASK USED?

It is essential to use the proper procedures for donning and doffing his mask. Be careful not to touch your eyes, nose, and mouth when the cover is removed and wash your hands immediately afterward.

Here is a clear step by step guide to the best way to properly wear a face mask.

Important note: the CDC, masks "should not be placed in young children under two years old who has trouble breathing or is unconscious, incapacitated, or unable to remove the cover without help."

How to clean and disinfect cloth mask?

Only use dry masks when they get wet covers, even if only from breathing, which needs to be cleaned.

Masks regularly wash with detergent and regulate the machine cycles hot wash. Dry completely.

DIY fabric Surgical mask

Homemade cloth surgical mask to be

worn as a last resort in a crisis.

Materials

- ❖ cotton fabric, tightly woven
- ❖ 1/8 "elastic cords, or fabric
- ❖ Tools
- ❖ sewing machine and thread
- ❖ the scissors

rule

pins or sewing clips

Instructions

Cut the fabric. For an adult-sized mask, cut one rectangle of fabric 16 "long and 8.5" wide. Cut two elastics, each 7 "long. Or, cut four fasteners fabric 18" long.

For a mask size child, cut one rectangle of fabric 14 "long and 6.5" wide. Next, cut two pieces of elastic, each 6 "long. I am sewing the upper side with a pocket opening. Fold the fabric in two, with the right-side face.

Sew along the 8.5 "wide edge using an 8/5" seam allowance. Leave a 3 "opening at the center of the seam to create an opportunity for the filter sock, and to enable the mask to be rotated to the right after sewing.

Sewing along both sides of the seam of a sharper

edge.

Pin elastic fabric or tie. Pina flexible member on each side of the mask, from one end to the apex angle and one end to the corner of the bottom. If you use cloth ties, pin a knot at each corner, with the rest of the knot sandwiched inside two layers of fabric.

Sew side. Sew the hands of the face mask backstitch on the elastic ties or fabric for secure.

Cut corners, turn right on the mask, and press with an iron.

Sew Pleated

Create three evenly spaced 1/2 "folds. Pin the folds in place, making sure all the creases are in the same direction. Sew each side to secure the folds.

Note: when the mask is worn, pleats are open downwardly to prevent the collection of particles in the folding pockets.

Some hospitals are applying for an opening of the large pocket for filter changes faster - 4 "deal.

For a small size child, start with a square that is 6.5 "by 14".

For a big kid size, start with a square that is 7.5 "by 15."

Recommended products

Colour scissors sewing pins 250 pieces of glass ball quilting pins Headpins jewelry decoration dressmaker

Brother Quilting Machine, CS7000i, 70 stitches built

2.0 "LCD screen, table width, including ten sewing feet.

Brother Quilting Machine, CS7000i, 70 stitches built 2.0 "LCD screen, table width, including ten sewing feet.

Dritz 9330W braided elastic, White, 1/4 inch by 3-Yard

He did this project?

A free pattern for sewing surgical masks home for hospitals. Make a pleated mask series with a filter pocket and elastic ear loops or loops woven fabric or cotton T-shirt material.

Remember, before you start sewing a massive lot of masks, please call the hospital or clinic and make sure you both want and can accept homemade masks.

This week, give it to Dr. Hoda Kardooni again, which investigated the science behind medical masks, respiratory masks, N95 masks, and fabric. As highlighted in this article, you will discover strict protocols to follow if you want a cover to work effectively.

There is much debate in progress on a face mask for public use. At this challenging time, it is understandable that people are desperately looking for anything that can help protect against the pandemic however vaguely either using the mask or believe the assertion of any news agency randomness concerning a specific drug or dietary regimen

Some common themes emerge in this debate. We will review and discuss these based on available data and scientific sources points.

Why not teach people how to wear a mask properly?

But countries, where people wore masks, had a better result in controlling the epidemic!
Masks can stop transmission of asymptomatic infected individuals and pre-symptomatic.
Mask medical/surgical for health facilities
Medical masks (e.g., N95) and surgical masks are crucial for physicians and nurses' frontline. Protection of workers' health (personal health) infection is crucial to the fight against the pandemic effectively. Medical masks are appropriate for most cautions in the air are in health centers (rather than daily use), and there are dedicated specific guidelines and instructions on how to carry and fit correctly.

Explanation

Surgical masks are primarily designed to protect the environment from the user, while respirators are supposed to protect the user of the situation. However, these differences may not be apparent for non-medical personnel, so here's a brief description.

Surgical masks, also known as face masks or masks procedure, soft devices, folding, disposable creating a physical barrier between the mouth and nose of the user and the environment lose.

N95 respirators are respiratory protection devices designed to achieve a very close fit of the face, which is generally round and adapted to form a seal around the nose and mouth. It is essential to properly keep and wear N95 respirators for them to work effectively.

Medical masks have been shown to have a protective advantage on laboratory surgical masks. However, data are insufficient to determine conclusively whether N95 respirators are superior to surgical masks to protect health workers against communicable acute respiratory infections in healthcare settings.

Surgical masks and medical have strict protocols.

Indeed, studies show that the effectiveness of N95 respirators and surgical masks may be similar for the prevention of influenza. However, this may be because the N95 respirators are uncomfortable and tight, making breathing more difficult, which could lead to more frequent elimination than surgical masks.

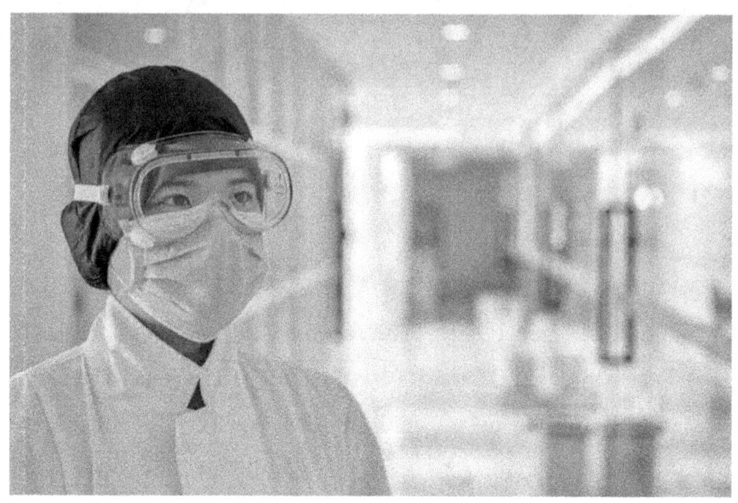

While the N95 respirators may confer superior protection in laboratory studies to obtain a 100% response accession, the systematic use of N95 respirators is less acceptable because they are single uncomfortable in practice. Therefore, these masks cannot be tightly molded to the face, which compromises the benefits of wearing an N95 respirator.

Masks domestic or community settings

If health care workers wear masks, should not the public as well? This debate has led to different policies worldwide.

The World Health Organization (WHO), the Center for Disease Control (CDC), and other public health resources have indicated that the only people who need to wear a face mask are those who are sick or take care of someone who is ill and unable to wear a mask Here, which confirms the above fact: Surgical masks (the easiest to get your hands on) designed to protect an infected person, further their structure enables them to capture body fluids excreted by the oral and nasal cavities (i.e., coughing and sneezing); however, they are not designed to protect the wearer against those infected.

Conversely, N95 masks, which are more challenging to obtain and more expensive to purchase, require specialized training to wear because they must be adequately molded to the wearer's face. Valid, the medical staff receive training and checking that they are adequately equipped.

Many contributing factors determine the effectiveness of masks:

Early use - before the infection is embedded at the location

adequate training - no training, users can not use the cover correctly

proper adjustment - the mask should not allow infectious particles in or outside Hand hygiene - unwashed hands may transfer infectious particles bearer the duration of costumes should be worn most of the time, not just when you go out In short, even if you have an N95 mask, there is a real possibility that this is not done correctly equipped and therefore, ensure optimal protection. So why are so many disagreements about this.

Why are the masks not as useful for the general public?

There is little data regarding masks to reduce the risk of infection at home or in the community.

There is ample evidence that health workers who are adequately trained in the use of masks and are exposed to a large number of infectious respiratory droplets are less likely to be infected.

20/03/2020-Coronavirus-pantryHow to store food for health during panic Coronavirus, However, a systematic review of published data (MacIntyre and Chughtai, 2015) reveals that masks do not prevent or reduce infection within the community when they are the only measure to prevent disease. The reason is that the effectiveness of masks is most likely affected by compliance issues.

There is consistent advice stressing that whether to wear a mask, you should use it appropriately.

This means:

- You should wash your hands before and after use or removal.
- Do not touch the front of it - the part exposed to infection.

- Avoid reaching down to scratch his nose or mouth.
- Use most of the time and discard as soon as it gets wet or damp.
- Otherwise, the use of masks could give a false sense of security.

It shows that compliance with these guidelines decreases in home settings with cover everyday use, which makes using a long-term challenge, In essence, this means that people become laxer about the correct use with time. This is particularly relevant in the current situation because the measures to suppress the spread of COVID-19 are necessary for long periods - not just a few days, but weeks and even months.

N95 masks must be appropriately fitted to work effectively

As noted by many studies, people did not adhere to keep the cover on all the time, simply because the 8uu6masks are uncomfortable. It is a difficult task to comply with all protocols that health workers are trained to routinely and implemented. For this reason, medical masks are recommended for the general public.

Why not teach people correctly use masks?

Teach people to wear a mask is not as easy as you teach them to wash their hands! It is complicated to wear a mask suitable even for health professionals who also are uncomfortable, but they have protocols to ensure compliance.

In addition to the lowest levels of compliance with the protocols of the mask in the home environment, many studies have found that people find less acceptable covers compared to hand hygiene behavior and other non-pharmaceutical interventions Countries using masks had better results in controlling the epidemic.

A recently circulated graph is comparing the mask wear-resistant countries (e.g., South Korea, Japan, Hong Kong, and Singapore) with states that did not ask the general public to wear costumes. The goal? To demonstrate that the wear-resistant mask is instrumental in suppressing COVID-19.

However, it is essential to note that many factors limit the spread of these countries, not only the use of masks. As you can see in the table below, many essential measures undoubtedly had more impact in controlling the spread and break the chain of transmission.

The factors that influence the spread of Covid-19

- strict social distancing quarantine
- cultural etiquette limiting physical contact
- the isolation of sufficient diagnostic tests for mild cases
- Also, several other essential facts have been omitted in this popular graphic. It does not include other countries, such as China, where face masks do not seem to have done much to spread Covid-19.
- Another example is Iceland, which is a remarkably well-controlled disease without the extensive use of face masks to the general public. Moreover, unlike the application, Singapore does not recommend universal covers and limit them to health workers.

The prevention of asymptomatic individuals to infect other

The transmission of symptomatic and asymptomatic individuals was documented pre-COVID for-19, and the viral load is particularly high in the early stages of the disease. This could make a case for wearing a mask as a public health intervention to intercept the transmission link.

DIY masks are not of medical grade protective equipment

However, we must keep in mind that even in

this situation, all the limitations arising from compliance with the cover are still valid. Also, if we assume that everyone is miraculously formed and adheres perfectly to all mask labels, there is still a big problem highlighted by the health authorities of the shortage of global supply chain of personal equipment protection (PPE) in hospitals worldwide.

Health workers have repeatedly reported the insufficient supply of PPE, ranging from gloves and protective gowns to wear goggles and face masks. Anyone who buys a cover for their use is potentially denying a health worker who needs it.

In this situation, there are two possible approaches to solve the problem:

masks home, but this requires technical knowledge of deep physics behind the filtration system tissues and medical masks.
Adhering to the measures based on evidence: washing hands, do not touch your face, physical distancing,

isolation of cases and quarantine.
Consider that this once again. Although a protective mask can reduce the risk of infection, it will not eliminate the risk, especially when the disease is more than one route of transmission. Thus,

any mask, no matter how active filtering or the quality of the seal, will have minimal effect if it is not used in conjunction with other preventive measures.

It is premature to assume that the masks protect people Covid-19 itself, and this could put the communities most at risk if you do not follow other strict protocols on how to use this mask and how to stay secure.

CHAPTER 6: PROBLEMS WITH A HOMEMADE MASK

To evaluate the use of a homemade costume, it is useful to know how the right cover (medical and surgical) work. Filtration systems used in modern surgical masks and respirators are considered "fibrous" in Nature: made of a flat, non-woven mat of fine fibers.

Every characteristic of the filtration system, including fiber diameter, porosity (ratio of open space to the fiber), and thickness, plays a role in how well the filter Koleksi particles. In all fibrous filters, three "mechanics" collection mechanisms are in place to capture particles, i.e., inertial impaction, interception, and diffusion.

You should wash your hands effectively even with a mask

inertial impaction and interception are the mechanisms responsible for collecting more massive particles, while diffusion is responsible for managing the smaller particles. In some fibrous filters made from fibers charged, an additional tool of electrostatic attraction also operates.

This mechanism helps in the collection of both large and small particles.

This latter mechanism is essential because it increases the particle collection without increasing the breathing resistance. Thus, the mask is not just a simple barrier, and there is more complexity in the cover work correctly, It is also important to note that the CDC, which is a list of homemade masks as an option for health care workers, also provides a choice of five alternatives to be used before switching to DIY:

Excluding health workers with a higher risk for severe illness from COVID-19 from contact with known or suspected COVID-19 patients.
Health workers recover designate (who already have the virus) for the treatment of known or suspected

COVID-19 patients.

Use a face shield that covers the entire front (which extends to the chin or below) and the side of the face without a facemask.
Consider using a prudent patient isolation room for patients at risk.
Consider the use of headrests ventilation in hospital beds to reduce exposure.

CDC Guideline has been developed for the use of masks in healthcare settings, so it is essential to understand that homemade masks are considered a last resort. They do not qualify as PPE since their protection capacity is unknown, and CDC urges caution when considering this option.

Many risks associated with cloth masks

cloth masks are commonly used in developing countries, and many non-standard practices regarding their cleaning and reuse have evolved. Most studies on the cloth masks were made before the development of disposable masks. Penetration through tissue is reported high. In one study, it was found that 40-90% of the particles can penetrate the cloth masks.

cloth masks allow more particles

A large prospective study RCT (Macintyre et al., 2015) showed that water retention, reuse cloth masks, and poor filtration could increase the risk of infection. They showed that the fabric masks have resulted in significantly higher rates of disease than medical masks, and worse than the controls.

fabric masks have given rise to higher infection rates

The virus can survive on the surface of cloth masks. Therefore, self-contamination by repeated use and improper doffing is possible (e.g., cloth mask contaminated pathogen can transfer cover with bare hands of the user).

cloth masks facilitate self-contamination

Although any material can be a physical barrier to infection, if it does not pass matches around the nose and mouth, or the material allows infectious particles to be free through it, it will be useless and dangerous.

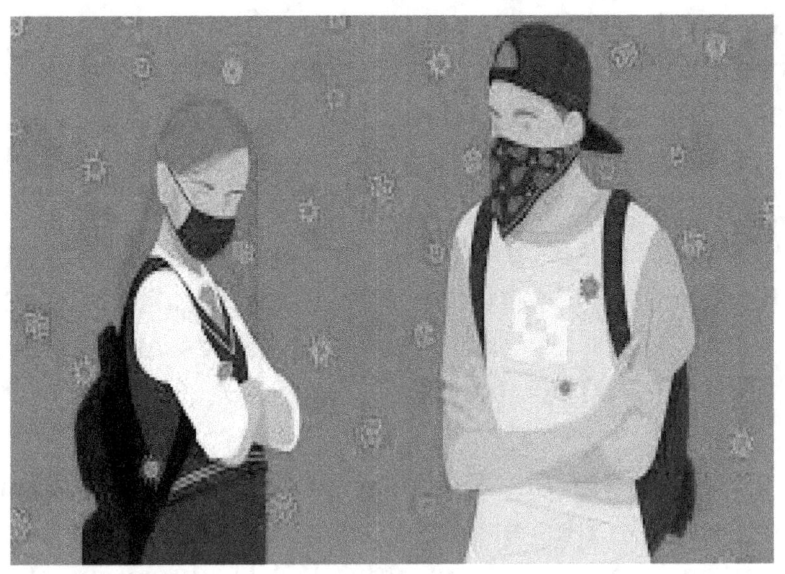

For those who wear a mask to the need, as health workers, regular training and fit testing must be emphasized. Those who choose to wear a mask homemade cleaning requirement must highlight the mask of the change. More importantly, it should be noted so that unnecessary risks are taken lower protective capabilities of a homemade costume.

What is a face mask for virus protection?

better-mask-protection against viruses

Although there are no masks that are specially

designed to protect against the infection alone, you can still find beneficial products that can filter viruses and other airborne particles. If you fear being infected with viruses, then you need to get masks that are approved by NIOSH and gave a rating of N95 or P100. It is those who have proven to be able to stop viruses mostly. You can say what masks are rated N95 or P100 because they are necessary to print detail on the cover itself.

If you do not find any indication of the mask dimension on the surface, or even on the box it came, then it is likely that it is not NIOSH approved at all. Apart from N95 and P100 masks, you can also use quality medical masks with high resistance to fluids. Ideally, they should be those who have resistance at three according to the ASTM standard.

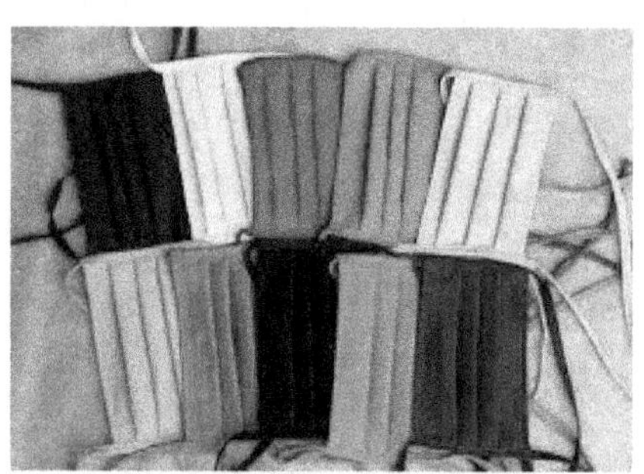

How does it work

Facial masks are air filters that you use on your face. The covers are made of non-woven. These fibers are trapped on the surface of a mesh static electricity charged. This creates a network of tiny holes arranged at random. This filter will provide a physical barrier between the outside air and the nose and mouth.

Masks work by blocking the harmful particles, including viruses, in which air into the nose or mouth. It's like a small network that traps tiny particles in the air, preventing them from getting into the nose and mouth.

The types of virus protection masks

There are many different types of facial masks that you can use to serve as protection against the virus. Here are some of the most popular options:

Medical Mask

This is the most common mask that people are using today. These look like pieces of paper with elastic bands on the sides that hook behind the ears. This form of respiratory protection is based on the filter material, which forms the entire mask.

The colored side of the mask is resistant to the liquid side. This is the part you want to be outside of if you're going to protect yourself from the disease. Now, if you are the one who has the flu, it is necessary
put the colored part of the inside of the mask.

Dust masks are disposable - This is the type of

cover which is generally used by craftsmen like carpenters, drywallers, carpenters, welders, and others who require respiratory protection. Note that these masks look like they are made of stiff paper.

However, the truth is that they are made of fibers which are joined together to create a fine mesh net, thereby preventing liquid and solid particles from getting through. A well as the masks medical/surgical, dust masks can be used only once. After that, then you should properly dispose of it. Never reuse this mask as its effectiveness and will have decreased by much.

Half-face respirators

These are the heavy-duty used for hazardous work environments. These have removable filters that are approved by NIOSH and rated N95 or P100 because they need to block the microscopic airborne irritants to the same asbestos fibers, glass fiber, silica, and others Do these masks be able to defend against viruses? Of course, they could. The only hindrance is that it will be disturbing when leads are out of the workplace. Also, they will be very intolerable to wear a whole sooner or later.

CHAPTER 7: WHY DO YOU NEED A FACE MASK FOR PROTECTION ANTIVIRUS?

The reason you need a face mask is that you can significantly reduce the chances of getting infected with the deadly disease when it comes to the outbreak of the virus. If your nose and mouth with a barrier that prevents aerosols are carriers of the virus to get through, then not be affected by them.

The way the virus is spread through coughing or sneezing of an infected person. The virus is carried in the saliva, and in the limited time that these particles are in the air if another person inhales, there is a good chance that they will become infected with the disease themselves

From now on, the virus is not airborne but has a limited distance you can travel. Besides wearing a mask, you should practice good personal hygiene also. You need to keep your hands clean because you may unknowingly touch a surface covered by the virus. This could put you at risk of touching the eyes, nose, or mouth with the virus, which leads to you getting the dangerous disease.

When it is your health that is on the line, you must ensure that the mask you buy can provide you with enough care and protection you need. Here are some things you should keep an eye on to purchase a good cover designed to protect you from viruses:

Stability

The first and foremost reason why you are considering buying masks is that you want to protect yourself and your family from being infected with the deadly virus circulating now. That is why, whenever possible, you should get one that is listed in the approved face mask CDC.

Now, it is understandable that people due to panic buying masks in bulk, most things in the CDC's list could be out of stock. If that is the case, then you should get one that is NIOSH approved and rated N95 or P100. These were most likely to block harmful particles in the air, which also happens to include bacteria.

Comfort - Many might think that comfort is not essential for masks, but it is. Even if you are dead serious about wearing your protective mask if, after an hour, it becomes unbearably uncomfortable under the cover, you will not want to pay more.

This could also be the time when you start to get complacent and more prone to infection. A good mask should be so light you'll forget you're wearing after a while. Here too

should be a way for your exhaled breath out of the cover.

This will prevent the inside of the mask to warm and soft. Moreover, it will save you from recycling your breath, which means you will not breathe in the carbon dioxide you just exhale.

Another factor that can contribute to a level of comfort is the head strap used to hold the mask in place. It should be neither too tight nor too loose. It should provide just enough elasticity to keep the cover in place.

Type mask

As mentioned above, many types of covers can be used to protect against viral infection, and levels of protection they offer also vary.

First, there is what we call as the disposable mask. You can buy this disposable type bulk for pennies each. The level of protection they offer is moderate at best, but if you're in a bind, you can expect that it is already working.

CHAPTER 8: THERE IS ALSO THE N95 MASKS OR REUSABLE P100.

These masks are much better protection against viruses, but they are a little more expensive. Also, you can use them for more than a day, but not by much. Most reusable masks can be used for about three days or until they get too dirty.

There are also bulky half-face respirators. They are those used by professional traders when they have to work in hazardous environments, such as when they must break down the walls and ceilings containing asbestos or must work with the delicate glass fiber.

Although these will give you more than enough protection, which is challenging to use in public and will also be very alarming to others.
Fit - Regardless of the type chosen, a good mask should fit properly on your face. There should be no space along the sides that allow outside air to enter into the cover. This contradicts the goal of bringing the mask in the first place.

An excellent way to know if there is a gap between the mask and the face is wearing glasses with the cover. If the windows fog at the exhaling,

there is a gap around the mask's nose.
To close this gap, pinch the metal band on the mask found on the bridge of the nose so it will take the shape of your nose. This will close the gap at the top of the cover.

Duration of use - Medical masks and dust masks are usually only just one use. Medical covers are only usable for three to four hours. If you feel that the inside is already wet, then you need to dispose of it immediately.

There are also reusable masks. Generally, are those exhale valves. Depending on the brand and the brand, you will often find a good cover for at least three days to a week.

Then there is the professional level. These are masks that can be reused indefinitely. Simply replace the filter cartridges once they are full. Most of the covers fall into this category are large and bulky and would look weird when used in public.

However, you can also find some of them seem regular facial masks but small cartridge filters/pads.

Cost and quantity - If you are thinking of buying a disposable type mask, you should ensure you get the most out of your money, literally. Disposable masks, such as medical masks, are cheap enough unless the seller jacks up the price due to increased demand, which is certainly unethical.

This does not mean you should get the cheapest out there. It is because you cannot be sure of its quality. You should buy masks that are sure of massively quality. This is because they are usually cheaper that way. A box of 100 masks can be much more expensive than a six-pack. When you do the math, you will find that the box 100s has a much lower unit price. Besides, the shape of things at this time, you may need to use facial masks for a long time, so it is best to have a lot in stock.

If you want something that is on the side of high strength and is worthy of being put in the survival kit of any person, payable over a hundred dollars for a full-face or half-face respirator.

Care and maintenance

If you are using disposable masks, you should immediately dispose of them at the end of the day. Never reuse disposable masks, especially surgical masks.

Also, if your medical mask gets wet, dispose of it immediately and use a new one instead. Another thing to consider is that when you start to feel that the cover is already humid, it is no longer usable.

Typically, all disposable masks, regardless of whether medical or dust masks need to be discarded after a day of use. Reuse is likely to get you infected if any viruses are trapped on the surface of the cover.

You must have masks properly. First, place them in a plastic bag, tie it, and put it back in the tray of hazardous waste. On the other hand, if you have a reusable mask, you should still have filter cartridges spending correctly and adequately clean the cover itself.

Most reusable masks are made of silicone, so they are straightforward to clean. There is only wiped with a solution made of equal parts of water and alcohol, and you're done.

CONCLUSION

This booklet us know the usefulness of wearing and non-wearing of a mask. Although it may be beneficial when the carrier is adequately trained on how to use and adheres to all other mask labels, there are other measures to protect against the spread of the virus and the risk behind it. Wash your hands, do not touch your face, and practice physical distancing.

DIY HOMEMADE MEDICAL FACE MASK

INTRODUCTION

This database project base on the impact of COVID-19 in the world economy drawer medical mask with a single step, giving us more information about creating a cover, and the gap between the traveler and the people go on holiday.

The development of this book is to give people a better understanding of the impact of COVID-19 in the world and to overcome the challenges against this crisis, which have affected the world economy in general and have had a negative effect.

CHAPTER 1: 7 WAYS TO MAKE A CREATIVE FACE MASK

1. HOW TO MAKE A FACE MASK WITH A SOCK

Then we'll show you how to make a face mask with a sock in less than a minute, which we think is quite ideal if you are looking for an affordable alternative to buying a facial mask. All you need is a single sock (preferably clean) and a pair of scissors.

When it comes to making a facial mask, this method is undoubtedly one of the easiest (and one of our favorites). After all, most of us have a strange stalking sock at the bottom of our drawer mysteriously partner anywhere.

How to successfully perform a mask using a sock, follow these steps:

1. Take a clean sock and cut along the hose's width, a couple of inches below the heel.

2. Cut along the length of the sock, on the opposite side of the heel.

3. Bend your longitudinal hose, so that the top of his sock meets in which he made the first cut.

4. create a small incision on the fold line - this should be only a couple of centimeters long. You should find that you have created two small slits on both sides of the mask - these loop around the ears.

5. Try in the mask size, using the heel of the sock over the nose. For an additional layer of protection, we have seen many people place a folded part on paper towels inside his mask.

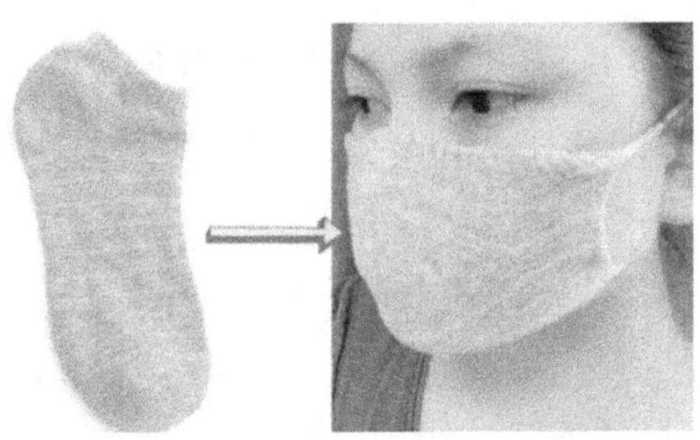

2. MAKING A FACE MASK WITH AN OLD T-SHIRT

Besides how easy it is to do, we also like the fact that you could just pop your shirt in the wash after a trip out to ensure adequate disinfection. This would reduce the risk of infection wearing masks.

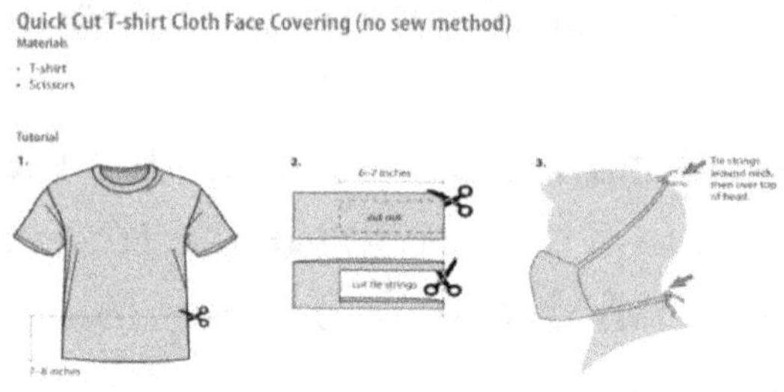

3. HOW TO MAKE A FACE MASK WITH A HANDKERCHIEF

This DIY mask without seams video tutorial could be the easiest we've seen. It is not only comfortable but fast, which means you can put your mask together in a minute or two if you are in a hurry.

All it requires is a handkerchief (a scarf or cloth large kitchen folded onto itself diagonally probably work well) and a pair of headbands.

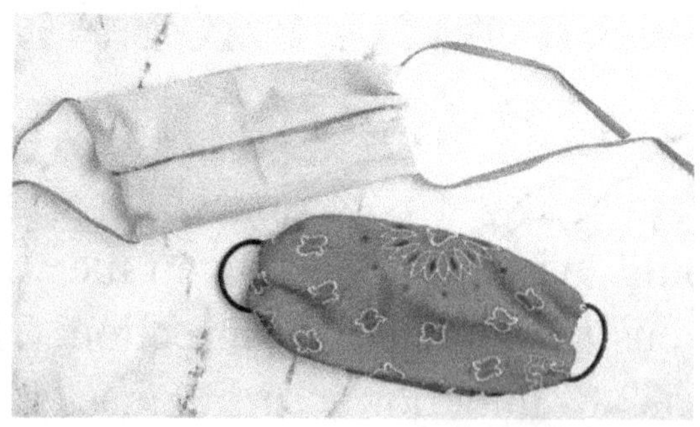

4. HOW TO MAKE A FACE MASK WITH A SCARF INFINITY

Infinity scarves are a better option worth considering if you are DIY-ing a face mask. It consists of lots of thin layers of fabric that can be wrapped tightly to your face without it becoming uncomfortable.

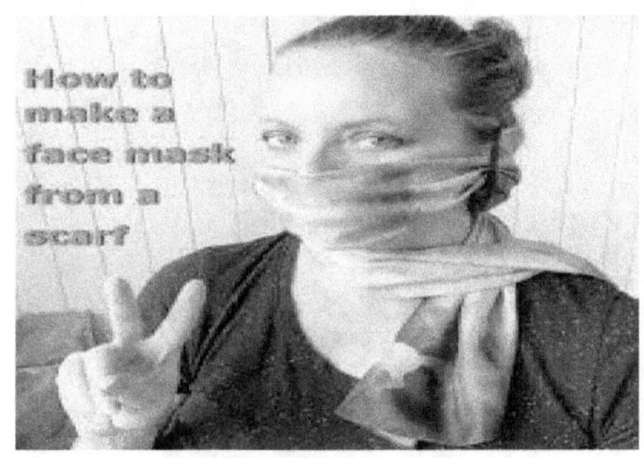

5. HOW TO MAKE A FACE MASK WITH A BUFF

While, unfortunately, none of us are going skiing in the short term, we might consider using an amateur like a face mask. We thought it might be one of the best choices if you are choosing to use a scarf as a makeshift mask.

They are very tight, which means you will not have to worry about crashing, but not restrict your breathing, because they are lightweight. Also, you can roll up to create multiple layers, which is similar to the approach we have seen applied to achieve many of the above options seamless.

You can also wash them in hot water wash, and will not lose its shape. They come in lots of colors and patterns, which can also be more attractive to children who are intimidated by the idea of wearing a face mask.

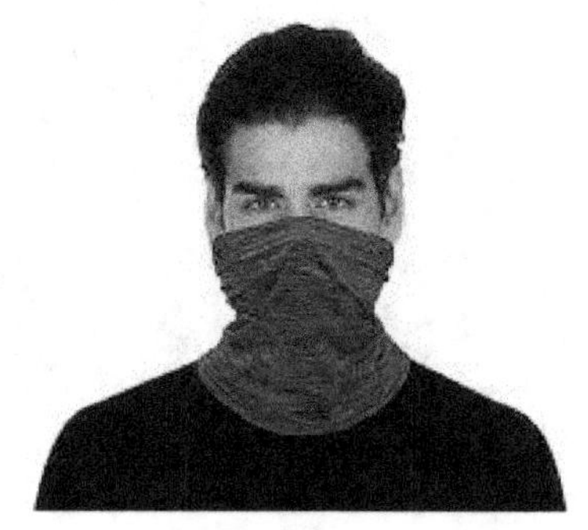

6. MAKING A MASK AND HEADBAND COMBO

Finally, this DIY mask without double seams like a headband, for example, I was walking to the store on the street with few people and only wanted to use his mask once inside.

The reason the mask is a social impulse

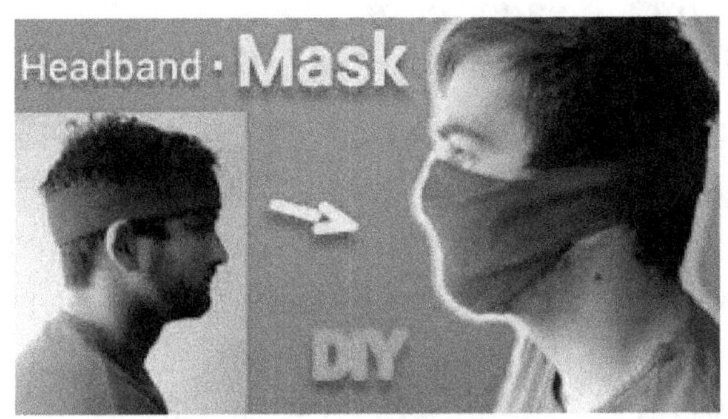

7. HOW TO MAKE A FACE MASK WITH SEWING MACHINE

1. Cut the fabric. For an adult size mask, cut one fabric rectangle 16″ long and 8.5″ wide. Cut two pieces of elastic, each 7″ long. Or, cut four fabric ties 18" long.
2. For a child-size mask, cut one fabric rectangle 14″ long and 6.5″ wide. Then, cut two elastic pieces, each 6 "long.
3. The upper side with an opening of the pocket. Fold the fabric in half, right side up.
4. Stitch along the 8.5 "wide edge, using a 5/8" seam. Leave a hole 3 "in the center of this seam to create so that the filter bag an opportunity, and to allow the mask is right side after sewing.

5. Press seam open. Zigzag along both sides of the suture by a cleaner edge.
6. Elastic tie pin or gender. Pin flexible piece on each side of the mask, an end at the upper corner, and one end to the bottom. When using tissue ties, pin a knot at each corner, with the rest of the lace sandwiched within the two layers of fabric.
7. Sew side. Sew the hands of the face mask—backstitch on the elastic ties or fabric for secure.

Cut corners, turn right on the mask, and press with an iron.

8. Sew Pleated Create three folds 1/2 "evenly spaced. Pin the folds in place, ensuring that all the creases are in the same direction. Sew each side to secure the folds.

Note: when the mask is worn, pleats are open downwardly to prevent the collection of particles in the folding pockets.

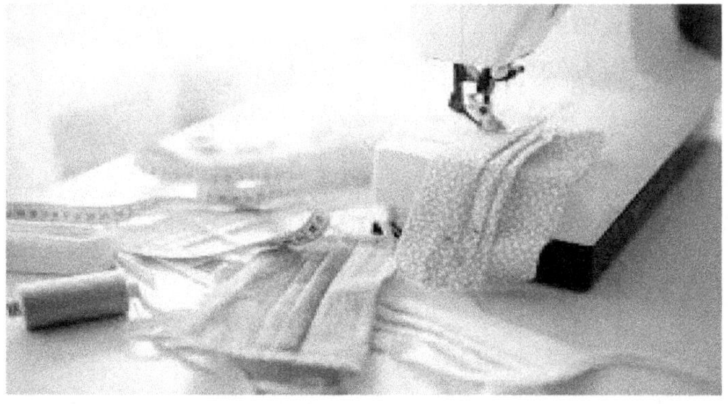

CHAPTER 2: THE REASON WHY THE FACE MASK IS A SOCIAL BOOST

WASHINGTON, DC - orientation of public health officials on how to avoid exposure to the new coronavirus has evolved over the crisis in the U.S.

Initially, counseling focused on handwashing, but more recently, authorities have urged Americans to wear face masks or covered in public. Consequently, an increasing number of Americans have adopted the use of masks to try to combat the spread of COVID-19. However, two recent studies by the Foundation Gallup / Knight show the new council seems to have introduced some confusion about the reasoning behind the recommendation to wear face coverings in public.

In late February, at the initial stage of the outbreak, U.S. Surgeon General Dr. Jerome Adams implored Americans stocking up on masks, saying they are not effective in preventing the general public from catching the disease and the need to be saved for health workers on the front lines.

Along with the US Centers for Disease Control and Prevention (CDC), Adams encourages the public to wash their hands often and thoroughly change. In

March, 88% of Americans said handwashing is more effective than surgical masks using, most of the rest (11%) saying that they were equally effective.

But on April 3, the CDC backtracked on its guidelines for face, following growing evidence that symptomatic and asymptomatic carriers R.P. can transmit the virus more quickly than previously thought. The new recommendation called for the use of masks or face cloth covers for Americans when and unable to follow the patterns of social distancing to prevent the spread to others, including unknowingly infected carriers in public.

The Gallup poll 14-20 / April Knight Foundation finds a sharp drop in the percentage of American adults who say hand washing is more efficient at 68%, and a concomitant increase in the rate that says handwashing and the use of masks are equally valid.

While changing patterns have introduced some confusion, the degree of change in all key demographic subgroups (including party identification, the communication media diet, and the amount of news consumption) is not substantial.

Notably, however, the opinions of older Americans are more likely to have changed. At the same time, younger adults remain hopeful that before I say handwashing is more effective in preventing wearing a mask.

Face mask habits of Americans

A separate survey question asked Americans how often they wore a mask covering the face or when they are in public in the last seven days. Those who have left their home in the previous seven days, on average to say he always wore a mask in general (36%), sometimes did (32%), and never did (31%).

In line with the findings of other surveys that ask about the face-covering Habits, Democrats, women, and people with higher education levels tend to say "always" or "sometimes" wore a mask over the last seven days.

Beyond these demographic differences, some other factors are correlated with the use of masks. For example, American adults who are users of heavy news, those who say they trust scientists and journalists "a lot", and those who live in a county that has recorded the deaths of at the least one of coronavirus related are more likely than their counterparts to say they always or sometimes wearing a mask in public in the last seven days.

In the same way, Americans who they think that wearing one is a mask as effective as hand washing in preventing healthy people from getting COVID-19 are more likely to say they had a face that covers the last seven days, compared to those who believe handwashing is more effective (75% vs. 66%).

Adhering to the CDC recommendation to wear masks is more evident among older Americans who believe that wearing a mask is as effective as hand washing.

bottom line

The American medical community's guidelines cover how Turnabout changed between March and April as new information emerged about the prevalence of symptomatic and asymptomatic P.R. and how the virus can spread.

The motivation behind the change in the orientation focused on preventing the spread of the virus by carriers. Still, the announcement has introduced some confusion about why people should wear masks.

Some members of the public seem to have falsely inferred that also implies that wearing a mask is an effective way to prevent healthy people from getting the disease. Yet there is no definitive scientific evidence to support or refute this.

Nevertheless, the announcement of these new guidelines was able to increase the use of masks in public spaces. Today, the majority of Americans say they always or sometimes wear a mask in public, especially those who consume a lot of new and trust the professionals such as scientists and journalists.

American social observation Remoteness less frequently.

Several states have begun to relax their social distancing guidelines regularly, while others have extended shelter requirements on site in May. Last week, 59% of Americans said that in the previous 24 hours, they "always" practicing social distancing. This is similar to 60% the last week but down from 65% reported that 6-12 April. Distancing percentage "very often" has not changed much, now at 29%, but the rate adhering less frequently increased by 7% to 12%.

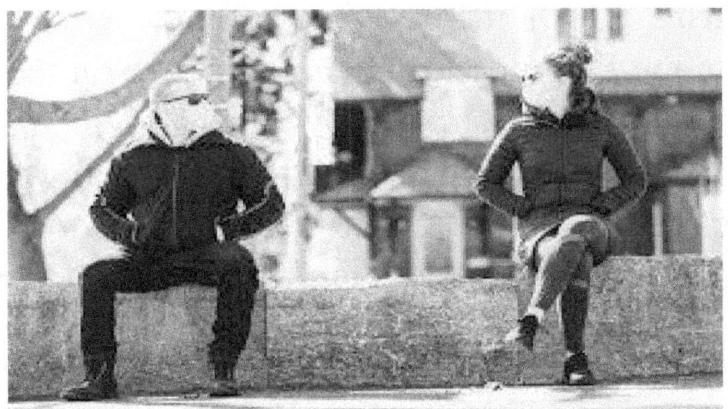

Most still avoid social situations in general.

At the least three-quarters of Americans, they say they have done each of the following components in the last seven days, while down slightly but still close to their April 30 March 5 senior Gallup interview.

86% avoided air travel and transit

80% avoided small gatherings of people, such as with friends and family

75% have avoided going to public places such as shops or restaurants

Also, 75% of Americans report now they have worn a mask on their face outside their home. This represents a 64% increase in the previous week and 51% in the first measuring Gallup, based on the 6-12 April interview. After joint discussion at the national level on whether the use of non-essential workers masks, April 3 the Centers for Disease Control officially recommended that almost all Americans wear cloth masks in public places where they cannot maintain social distancing guidelines.

CHAPTER 3: COVID-19 IMPACT ON THE WORLD ECONOMY

Since coronavirus spreads worldwide, states are grappling with finding the ideal strategy to address the global pandemic. In China, Singapore, South Korea, the U.S., the U.K., and Europe, different policies are a product of the State's capacity and the legal authority. Still, they also reveal competing views on the optimal role of centralized state authority, federalism, and the private sector.

While it is too early to know the long-term effects, the apparent ability of state authority centralized in China, South Korea, and Singapore to respond effectively and quickly made headlines in the U.S., the opposite was accurate.

The U.S. response is being shaped by its federal structure, a dynamic private sector, and culture of citizen participation. In the three weeks since the first U.S. case coronavirus, state leaders, public health institutions, companies, universities, and churches have been at the forefront of the efforts of the nation to mitigate its spread was confirmed.

Images security workers in hazmat suits disinfection offices of multinational corporations and university campuses populate the Facebook pages of America. The contrast with the efforts of the White House to manage the message, minimize, then quickly increase its estimate of the crisis is hard.

Puzzling response

For European viewers, the absence of a clear and focused response from the White House is puzzling. By the time Donald Trump President declared a national emergency, emergencies, and various State had was called, universities online learning had shifted, and churches began to close.

In contrast, in Italy, France, Spain, and Germany, the State directed national efforts to seal the borders and schools. In the U.K., schools are being opened primarily as prime minister. Boris Johnson has declared a defined strategy for herd immunity, which revolves around the exposure of populations resistant to the virus.

But the United States never shared the belief in Europe that the State should lead. The Centers for Disease Control and precaution., the leading national public health institute, and a federal U.S. agency have tried to establish a benchmark for the assessment of the crisis and advise the nation. But in this case, their response has been delayed due to flaws in the initial tests it came to deployment. The Federal Reserve has moved quickly for cutting interest rates and cut them back further this week.

But states were the true pioneers in the response of the United States. They had been using his authority to declare a state of emergency independent of the declaration of a national emergency. This has enabled countries to mobilize critical resources and the cities of pressure in action. After several days of delay and intense public pressure, the governor of New York, Andrew Cuomo, forced New York Mayor Bill de Blasio to close schools in the city.

State emergency declarations by individual states have given companies, universities, and churches the freedom and legitimacy to run and be ahead of the federal government to stop the spread in their communities.

Washington State was the first to declare a state of emergency. Amazon, one of the largest employers in the country, quickly announced a halt to all international and travel, and Microsoft, who donated $ 1 million to fund rapid emergency response based in Seattle. United have pushed their corporations to pioneer the response coronavirus sector. However, companies have voluntarily adopted the challenge, often getting ahead of state and federal action.

Google rushed to announce a move that allows employees to work from home after California declared a state of emergency. Facebook soon followed with an even stricter policy, insisting employees work from home. Both companies have also met with the World Health Organization (WHO) officials to discuss responses and predictable funding for the Solidarity Response Fund established WHO in collaboration with the Foundation U.N. and the Swiss Philanthropy Foundation.

Leading research universities in the U.S., with a unique position in the local public health and legal experience, have also been boosting prevention efforts. Explains just days after Washington, a state of emergency, the University of Washington was the first to announce the end of teaching in the classroom and online courses movement. A similar pattern followed in Stanford, Harvard, Princeton, and Columbia - each also following the declaration of a state of emergency.

Moreover, the Church of Latter-day Saints' decision to cancel their services worldwide continued declaration of a state of emergency Utah.

The hole in the U.S. response It has been the national government. President Trump's declaration of national emergency arrived late, and his decision to ban travel to Europe, but initially excluding the

U.K., created uncertainty and concern that politics as much unity of the response of the House white as evidence.

This may change soon, as the House of Representatives has approved a bill COVID-19 response that the Senate will consider. These movements are vital to support public and private efforts to mobilize an effective response to a national and global crisis.

Need for public oversight

In the absence of better coordination and leadership of the center, the U.S. response it pales in comparison to China's dramatic moves to stop the spread. Chaos at airports in the United States shows the need for public oversight. As New York State Governor Cuomo declared the support of the federal government to build new hospitals, he said: 'I can not do it. It cannot be left to the states.

When it comes to global pandemics, we can discover that authoritarian states may have a short-term advantage. However, Iran's response and demonstrates that this is not the universal case. Eventually, registration of all authoritarian states as they tackle the coronavirus will become more evident and is likely to be mixed.

Open societies remain essential. Prevention requires innovation, creativity, the free exchange of information, and the ability to inspire and mobilize international cooperation. The State is undoubtedly necessary, but not sufficient by itself.

Efforts and resources of the State Department

The team of the State Department is working tirelessly to fight start

The State Department is taking decisive action to inform and protect U.S. citizens abroad, protect the homeland, promote the Administration's commitment to build global health security for this and future outbreaks, and reduce the impact on the U.S. companies and supply chains abroad.

We advise U.S. citizens to avoid all international travel due to the global impact of COVID-19.

Protecting the Homeland

The priority of the Department is to protect the United States and curb the spread of the virus. We have implemented travel restrictions prudent, together with our interagency partners, for people who have been present in areas considered high risk by health authorities in the United States. Traveling to protect U.S. citizens or live abroad, continually updated our travel warnings and alerts timely issuance of country-specific commuters to keep Americans informed and safe third.

Keeping U.S. Informed citizen travelers

The Department uses a wide range of instruments, including travel reviews and alerts to communicate the apparent security, fast, reliable, and safety information to help American citizens to make informed decisions about travel abroad. Every American embassy and the consulate has also updated its website to U.S. citizens in all countries of the world who have access to the latest details on Covid-19. We will continue to update this information frequently and encourage the United States.

Citizens read our latest opinions travel in their entirety and to register for receiving further updates Register Smart Traveler Program (STEP.state.gov).

Supporting the Labor Ministry and the preparation of our employees

The security and safety of our workforce are to departmental priorities. The ministry has issued interim guidelines on flexibilities leave and work for employees ordered or authorized departure and will update this advice is needed.

As a precautionary measure, the Department requested posts abroad to call their emergency action committees (CEC) to ensure the respective preparation after. The Office of Medical Services follows the recommendations of the CDC and WHO regarding the prevention, diagnosis, isolation, and treatment of all infectious diseases.

Support the response of the U.S. government

Assistant Secretary of State Stephen Begun directs the U.S. Department for his efforts on the White House coronavirus working group that coordinates and oversees the Administration's efforts to monitor, prevent, contain, and mitigate the spread of the virus. Experts from across the Department were mobilized by leveraging a wide range of stakeholders from the private sector bilateral, multilateral, and partners for a response consular, diplomatic, economic, and regional synchronized global Coordinating Unit Response coronavirus (CGRCU).

CHAPTER 4: OUR GLOBAL HEALTH LEADERSHIP

The White House appointed head of global health world-renowned physician and Ambassador Deborah Birx in the office of the Vice President with the whole of government response to Covid-19 as coordinator of coronaviruses interventions. Dr. Birx is exceptionally well equipped for this role, given his years of experience to lead the worldwide fight against HIV / AIDS as head of the President's Emergency Plan for the fight against AIDS Relief (PEPFAR).

Bring Home the Americans

Embassy Panama City staff work to help American citizens who return home on April 2, 2020. [State Department Photo / Public Domain]

The State Department increases to meet the critical challenge posed by the pandemic Covid-19, every day, everywhere.

The U.S. government has no excessive prime concern than protecting U.S. citizens. The State Department has launched a global effort to bring unprecedented citizens from all corners of the international and has repatriated thousands of

Americans from several countries. Our organization is working around the clock in Washington and abroad, bring home thousands more in the coming days, from all regions of the world.

Helping U.S. citizens around the world

We perform to ensuring the safety of U.S. citizens abroad. In an exceptional effort, we repatriated tens of thousands of people in the United States in response to the epidemic Covid-19, in close coordination with the CDC and HHS public health experts. We continue to advocate U.S. citizens use commercial travel options and follow the advice of local authorities. We will continue working with our international partners to fight against the epidemic, help those who remain abroad and minimize risks for our citizens worldwide.

International Aid and Relations

President Trump's leadership, thanks to the generosity of the American people, has continued to demonstrate its international leadership in public health and humanitarian assistance in the face of the pandemic COVID-19. The management is deploying the full range of U.S. resources to contain and prevent the spread of COVID-19 at home and around the world.

Since the outbreak of COVID-19, the U.S. Government has committed more than $ 1 billion in foreign aid to date. This funding will improve public health education, health centers protect and increase laboratory, disease surveillance and rapid response capacity in more than 120 of the riskiest in the world of all countries to help contain the outbreaks before they reach our shores.

The State Department, USAID, and CDC are working together to support systems for health, humanitarian and economic assistance, security and stabilization efforts worldwide with $ 2.4 billion in charge of emergency funds Congress has appropriated.

The United States is by far the most generous and reliable partner to respond to the crisis and humanitarian action through UNICEF, the World Food Program, and many international organizations. Our leadership enables these organizations to combat the disease and, ultimately, protect Americans.

Americans not only assists with government media. We've helped populations affected by the pandemic COVID-19 around the world through the generosity of private companies, nonprofit groups, and faith-based organizations.

The United States has always stood by our partners through pandemics and crises. In the face of the COVID-19, the American people are here to help.

Collaboration with partners and allies

The Department is actively working with international partners and governments to combat the spread of the outbreak. Reaffirming the importance of diplomacy every step of the way, we have maintained close communication and close coordination with the countries concerned and implements the U.S. Government restrictions or problems advisory updates to ensure the necessary travel bilateral relations remain stable in the face of prudent and robust public health measures. The Government has informed the U.S. more than 100 officials from more than 70 nations.

We are also working with international public and private sector partners, including WHO, to rapidly improve our knowledge about the virus, our public health decisions, and accelerate research and development of vaccines, therapeutics, and diagnostics.

Building Global Health Security for the first line

The Department shares a global interest in the prevention, detection, and response to infectious disease threats at the source. The Department continues to promote the security agenda of the Global Health (GHSA) and coordinate the implementation of activities that help strengthen laboratories. Diagnostic equip front-line workers with the necessary tools and stocks to protect against outbreaks emerging, including this coronavirus (COVID-19) outbreak. These associations have laid the groundwork to prepare quickly and effectively to emerging threats, including COVID-19. Investments in global security of U.S. health are one of the most effective ways to save lives and protect U.S. citizens from global pandemics and the spread of pathogens.

Mitigate the impacts International Business USA

The White House, the Department, and other government agencies are coordinating U.S. provide U.S. companies and employers with information about COVID-19. The Administration is monitoring the possible effects of COVID-19 supply chains and summon the pharmaceutical companies' leaders on the challenges of the supply chain that could affect the United States.

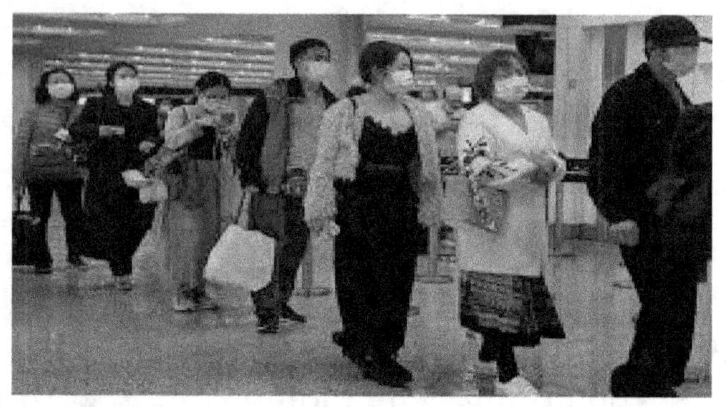

Promoting Transparency

The United States remains deeply concerned about information indicating that some government schemes may have suppressed vital details about the outbreak and, given the implications for public health, continues to reiterate that all countries transparently share information and cooperate with public health organizations and relevant international help.

The Centers for Disease Control and Prevention said Friday he had been mixing the test results of viral antibodies and on its website. The CDC says it is planning to separate those numbers in the coming weeks, but experts say that the current method is useless and potentially misleading.

This is because no antibody tests are used to diagnose a current infection or determine whether a person is potentially infectious. Instead, they indicate whether someone has been exposed to the virus in the past.

CDC spokeswoman Kristen Nordlund describes the practice of the agency told CNN on Thursday and confirmed the next day. "At the beginning, when CDC launched its much more common nationwide website and its reports laboratory test, viral tests (current infection) is used to serology tests (evidence of past infection)," he said an email.

"Now that serology tests more widely available, CDC is working to differentiate those tests for viral testing and report this information, differentiated by the type of test, published on our website COVID Data Tracker in the coming weeks."

Several pulses of antibodies and viral testing are combining up to the total number of experiments carried out in the USA. However, antibody tests are often intended for the general public - not just people with suspected infections - so it can skew a crucial indicator of how the pandemic is progressing: the percentage of positive tests.

CDC method also makes it appear that the U.S. has a higher capacity to test what it does, at least when it comes to identifying current infections.

"There is useful information unless you have a political agenda that you are trying to back up. That's the only reason to do that," he told CNN Medical Analyst Dr. Celine Gounder, professor of medicine and infectious diseases at the NYU School of Medicine.

CHAPTER 5: WHAT IS THE IMPACT OF CORONAVIRUS ON ECONOMY?

The impact of the coronavirus in the confidence of European companies remains limited.

Later this week will hit confidence figures for the Chinese economy for February.

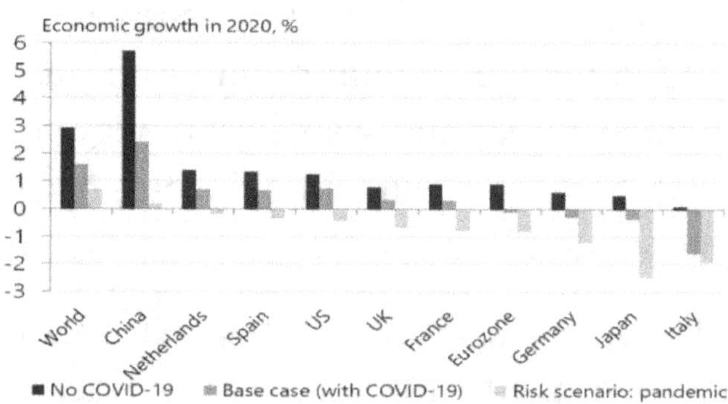

American consumers should continue to spend, and that's what we're planning.

Gold prices last week reached its highest level since March 2013. Traditionally, gold has performed well in times of uncertainty. The coronavirus causes the latter.

The rate at which the virus spreads appears to be declining slowly, but the epidemic is not yet content, much less. New cases in Italy testify to this. We also have to see what will happen if the Chinese, at some point, to return en masse to work. Meanwhile, more and more companies undoubtedly supply problems and report production.

In any case, the first quarter of 2020 can be considered "lost" growth. China within a likely economic contraction compared to the last quarter of 2019, and worldwide growth halved.

The words of the President of Trump only add to the confusion She had told him last week that his reassurances were contradictory with prevention messages federal health authorities. This confusion in the letters of Washington has been pointed out by Democrats. Donald Trump accused of a hoax. When is the press that the questions themselves, denouncing the hysteria?

However, he continues. For example, recently gave a telephone interview with FOX News, the most-watched, three and a half million people s and their statements were then widely distributed.

Words truly amazing. First, he disputes the mortality rate of the WHO, and he said that these figures are wrong and that the virus kills far less than the claims of the World Health Organization. And to justify this charge, it is said to be his "hunch."

The President also believes that for many patients, the virus will be very smooth. And even he says better have to go to work. This is contradictory to the warning messages sent by the authorities, who recommend not going to work if you have symptoms. Donald Trump still obtained from Congress the release of more than $ 8 billion to deal with the crisis.

Coronavirus has little impact on the confidence of European business.

China PMI will scare the markets?

Next weekend, the office of Chinese official statistics (NBS) released its PMI (business confidence, measured by purchasing managers). These fully reflect the disorders associated with coronavirus. The fact is known, but it remains to be seen whether financial markets were spooked even more.

When investments go up?

In the U.S., we have paid particular attention to the willingness to invest in companies for a while. He played in a minor key. This was confirmed, for example, by small recent figures for loans in the industry. However, investments are essential if we want to achieve, as expected, about 2% economic growth for all of 2020.

On Thursday, we will receive the figures for durable goods orders for January. These figures are also an indication of the demand for capital goods. In recent months, new capital goods orders were below expectations. It will be a question of observing whether a turnaround is taking shape. Although, in this area too, coronavirus could (temporarily?) Confuse the issue.

We always count on the American consumer.

The U.S. consumer confidence seems to have been infected to date. This, of course, thanks to a stable job market and stock markets booming in recent weeks.

Dynamic spending nevertheless declined somewhat in the last quarter of 2019. Similarly, retail sales have been moderate in January. Perhaps because wage growth, despite labor shortages, remains limited. The average number of hours worked also seems to decrease somewhat.

Nevertheless, we still rely on the fact that Joe Six-Pack continues to support the U.S. economy. As investments - as stated above - do not restart, this support is particularly crucial. At the end of this week, personal income and spending for January will already give us an indication in this regard.

CHAPTER 6: THE IMPACT OF COVID-19 HAD ON TOURISM.

While the global financial crisis that began in 2007 in 2012 extends, its effects are felt everywhere: trust in banks slid, more families have no cash, and international migration is falling. Not unexpectedly, tourism has been affected as well, with a series of impacts at the national and international levels.

A 2010 report in The Journal of Research Travel, "The impacts of the global recession and economic crisis on tourism: North America," examines how the financial crisis affected Canada Travel, United States, and Mexico. The University of Colima, based on its report on multiple sets of data on tourism from 2004 to 2009.

In the USA:

In and in the United States, tourism has steadily declined in the year and a half after the 9/11 attacks. "In the six quarters advanced to the fourth quarter trough, the actual demand for travel fell by 9.5%. However, the real GDP of the nation increased by 1% during this period. "From that low point, the demand has grown at a rate of 3.7% per year to reach a new high in the third quarter of 2007. At the same time, the delayed real GDP growth at 2, 7% per year.

The current economic decline began in December 2007; in early 2009, the US GDP fell by nearly 4%, the worst drop since World War II.

In the first quarter of 2009, the actual demand for travel fell 6% over six quarters. "This decrease was far more gentle than what took place after the 9/11 attacks. But the decline was twice as fast as real GDP dropped.

"Tourism employment culminates at nearly 6 million jobs in the first quarter of 2008. Therefore, in the first quarter of 2009, more than 250,000 jobs were lost in the sector.

Even though the slight inflation continues, "travel prices have fallen twice as fast in the current recession as after the 9/11 attacks. "

In Mexico.

Despite natural disasters and ongoing issues with internal security from 2005 until the first half of 2008, international arrivals to Mexico rose to nearly 6% per year. However, there was a remarkable variation along the way, including drops of 5.35% in 2006 and 3.9% in 2007.

"The data [confirm] that there are other factors that have a major impact on the tourism industry in Mexico that the collapse of financial markets and economic activity."

The exchange rate between the peso and other currencies has a significant influence on the influx of foreign visitors. "Ironically, when the Mexican economy falters, and the peso depreciates, the benefits of the tourism sector and tourism services in Mexico are more affordable in the eyes of foreign visitors."

For Canada:

From 2007 to 2008, Canadian spending in the United States decreased by 15%, and spending the U.S. in Canada, declined by 6%.

In May 2009, international travelers made 1.4 million overnight trips to Canada, down 7% from the previous year.

Donald Trump said the United States would suspend all trips from Europe for 30 days from Friday.

Will Canada have to do the same with the United States?

The U.S. president said in a speech to the nation delivered Tuesday night.

The closure of the U.S. border, which will have significant consequences for the world economy, will be in effect from midnight on Friday. The United Kingdom is not affected by the measure.

Donald Trump has been attributed partly to blame Europe for the situation in his country, not to close their borders quickly to travelers from China or other countries affected by the virus.

At the moment, Canada is safe from this measure imposed by Trump. However, nothing is guaranteed, according to our columnist Bernard Ville drain.

A heavyweight

Most calculator's carbon footprint estimates that the use of a car adds about 2.5 tons of greenhouse gases for the balance of a person per 10,000 kilometers traveled. Leave your car at home to take public transportation can reduce the carbon footprint of a person by 26% to 76%, according to some studies.

"It is clear that the abandonment of the car is what has the most significant impact because it eliminates emissions due to the use of the vehicle, but also those linked to manufacturing, which is very important in terms of weight of carbon. 'A vehicle. This is why carpooling would be an effective solution, limiting the two sources of emissions associated with cars, more than carsharing, "adds MS Potvin.

Ineffective Gestures

Governments are multiplying campaigns and guides to encourage citizens to reduce their carbon footprint. However, according to a study conducted in 2017 at the University of Vancouver and the University of Lund in Sweden, most of the proposed actions by public officials are successful for relatively ineffective measures oriented to reduce greenhouse gases. Tight.

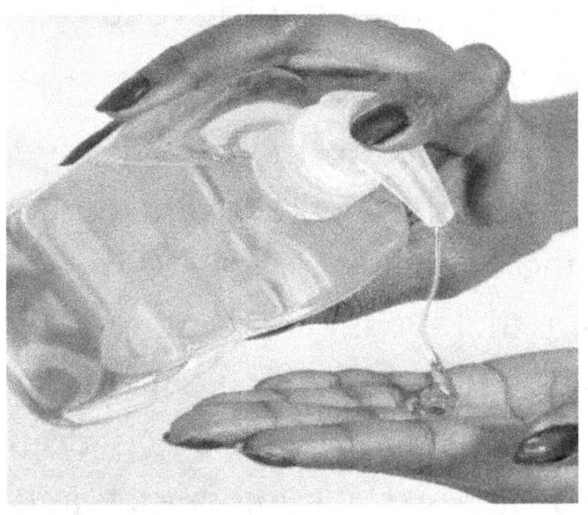

More than 148 proposed actions, the three countries with the carbon footprint highest per capita in the world (Canada, United Kingdom, and the United States), none suggests reducing air transport (between 0.7 and 3.2 tones of CO2 per flight) or the benefits of a meatless diet (a discount of up to 1.6 tons per year).

Furthermore, various measures guides include a low impact on greenhouse gases, such as drying clothes to the outside (-0.21 tCO2 / yr) or the laundry in cold water (-0.25 tCO2 / year) more efficient measures to reduce your electricity bill gases associated with global warming.

Beneficial and direct solutions are often absent from public discourse, Catherine Potvin believes.

Instead of adopting a guilty tone for the use of motorized transport, she said, she must promote solutions to avoid avoidable trips such as teleworking or Skype meetings.

"I think we need to look at other ways of doing things. We have the highest rate of emissions per person in the world, which seems to be reason enough to say that we have a long way to go. Indeed, in the regions, people often have no choice other than the car. And this is where governments must intervene. For the rest, it's like a diet, and we start by cutting where it hurts the least. "

It rings a new virus in China and rose to six dead, and more than 300 cases on Tuesday as millions of Chinese people are willing to travel for the Lunar New Year, which increases the risk of contagion.

Many in China are scrambling to buy masks to protect against coronavirus infection, such as influenza previously unknown and airports World tight screening.

The epidemic, which began in the central Chinese city of Wuhan, also concerned about the financial markets, investors recalled the economic consequences of a severe outbreak of severe acute respiratory syndrome (SARS) in China in 2002/2003 it initially covered.

The SARS coronavirus has killed nearly 800 people then.

"We will stay at home during the holidays. I'm afraid I vividly remember SARS, "said Zhang Xinyuan, which had been bound from Beijing to the Thai resort of Phuket before she and her husband definite to cancel their tickets.

Authorities confirmed more than 300 cases of new coronavirus in China, mostly in Wuhan, provincial capital and transportation hub, where it may come from a seafood market.

Manifestation includes fever, coughing and breathing difficulties, and viral infection can cause pneumonia.

Wuhan Mayor Zhou Xian Wang said Chinese state television Tuesday six people had died in his city. The disease is spreading around other parts of China, including five cases in the national capital Beijing.

"Fifteen medical personnel are among those illnesses."

Abroad, Thailand has reported two cases and South Korea, all involving Chinese Wuhan. Japan and Taiwan have confirmed one each incident, the two nationals who had been in Wuhan.

The World Health Organization (WHO) held a meeting on Wednesday to consider whether the epidemic is an international public health emergency.

Doctors and alarmed markets

"Information on new infections reported suggest it may be now sustained human transmission," said WHO Regional Director for the Western Pacific, Takeshi Kasai.

Taiwan, the island governed by saying that China claims as its own, set up an epidemic response center. Over 1,000 beds have been prepared in isolation wards in case the virus spreads further.

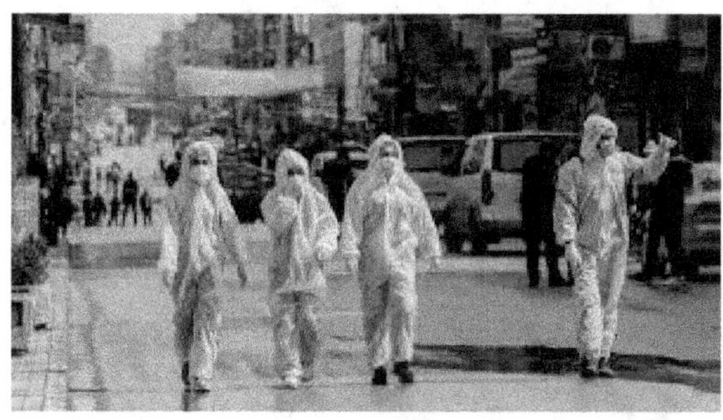

North Korea was to ban foreign tourists, who are mainly Chinese temporarily, an international tour operator said.

Fear agitated risk aversion in global markets, with Asia particularly affected.

Hong Kong, which has suffered much during the SARS outbreak, saw its index down 2.8%. Japan's Nikkei lost 0.9% and 1.7% blue-chip Shanghai, with the pressure airlines.

Coronavirus cases will increase as more people travel ahead of the Lunar New Year

In Europe, shares of luxury goods manufacturers, which have broad exposure to China, were among the most decline.

The Chinese yuan fell nearly 0.7% in offshore operations to 6.9126 per dollar, on land, which fell to its lowest level in more than a week at 6.9094.

Although the virus's origin has not yet been identified, WHO said it was probably the primary source of animal. Chinese officials have linked the outbreak of the Wuhan seafood market.

More functions and masks

"The outbreak of SARS coronavirus in Wuhan is becoming an important potential economic risk of the Asia-Pacific now that there is medical evidence of human to human transmission," said Rajiv Biswas, chief Asia Pacific economist at IHS mark it.

So far, WHO has not recommended travel restrictions or trade, but can be discussed on

Wednesday. National Health Commission of China is also scheduled to give an update at a press conference at 10 a.m. on Wednesday.

Airports in the United States, Australia, and Asia have begun screening passengers extra Wuhan.

In the city itself, officials have been using ruddy thermometers to screen travelers at airports, railway stations, and other traveler terminals from January 14.

The Lunar New Year is an important holiday for the Chinese, many of whom travel to join the family or have a holiday abroad.

Long lines formed to buy masks in cities. Some online vendors selling masks and hand sanitizers limited because of the increased demand.

According to the publication on the website of Shanghai Observer, market regulator Shanghai city warned that punish speculators hoard masks or other products used for the prevention of infectious diseases.

Chinese travel booking platforms from to Fliggy Alibaba Group said they would offer free cancellations in bookings made for Wuhan, while South Korea's low-cost airline Air T'way postponed the launch of a new route to the city.

Zhong Nanshan, head of the team of the National Health Commission investigating the outbreak, aimed to improve alarm, saying in images shown on state television that there was no danger that the SARS epidemic repeat, as long as they take the precautions.

T'Way launch air is stopped due to virus concerns.

Due to the growing concern about the spread of a new coronavirus, South Korea's low-cost airline Air T'way has postponed the scheduled launch Tuesday of a new route to the Chinese city of Wuhan.

Monday, South Korea reported the first confirmed case of the illness from 35-year-old Chinese national who flew from Wuhan to Seoul on Sunday.

T'way was set for the first of two times a week from the central axis of Korea South Incheon to Wuhan at 1020 pm (1320 GMT), but canceled plans because of the epidemic, and the official said the company.

"It was an unavoidable decision because of the situation there," the official told Reuters, adding that it will closely monitor developments.

The decision came amid spiraling fears about the virus, which could spread through human contact with millions of Asians traveling on vacation the Lunar New Year this week. In China, the number of confirmed cases rose to 291 on Monday.

An official of the Korean Air Lines, the only other airline Korean Southern direct flights to Wuhan works, said the company has no plans to suspend its route four times running per week, but not to raise cancellation fees Tickets for travel to the city,

Centers South Korea for Disease Control and Prevention warned on Tuesday tourists from contact with animals and people showing respiratory symptoms and visits market in China.

President Moon Jae-in instructed local authorities to step up prevention efforts, with many South Koreans living in China. He expected to return home and some 32 million traveling around the country for vacation until next week.

FASHION NOW

Too little or too much money? Here's what the IRS said about inaccurate stimulus payments

Mitch McConnell Senate majority leader, R-KY,

The following Bill coronavirus is a "final," said Mitch McConnell

Here's how the unpaid debt is processed when a person dies

Protesters burn a flag outside the CNN Center on May 29, 2020, in Atlanta, Georgia. Events are held across the U.S. after George Floyd died in custody on May 25 in Minneapolis, Minnesota.

Protests and riots in cities in the U.S. that the bubbling anger after the assassination of George Floyd

A prototype rocket SpaceX Starship after a test explosion on May 29, 2020.

SpaceX prototype explodes the Starship rocket after the test in Texas

by commercial tabula.

The results of a new virus in China rose to six dead, and more than 300 cases on Tuesday as millions of Chinese people were willing to travel for the Lunar New Year, which increased the risk of contagion.

Many in China are scrambling to buy masks to protect against coronavirus infection, such as influenza previously unknown and airports World tight screening.

The epidemic, which began in the central Chinese city of Wuhan, also concerned about the financial markets, investors recalled the economic consequences of a severe outbreak of severe acute respiratory syndrome (SARS) in China in 2002/2003 it initially covered.

Symptoms include fever, coughing and breathing difficulties, and viral infection can cause pneumonia.

Wuhan Mayor Zhou Xian-wang said Chinese State television Tuesday six people had died in his city. The disease is spreading around other parts of China, including five cases in the international capital Beijing.

Fifteen medical personnel are among those infected.

Abroad, Thailand has reported two cases and South Korea, all involving Chinese Wuhan. Japan and Taiwan have confirmed one each incident, the two nationals who had been in Wuhan.

The World Health Organization (WHO) held a meeting on Wednesday to consider whether the epidemic is an international public health emergency.

"It was an inevitable decision because of the situation there," the official told Reuters, adding that he would continue to monitor developments.

The move came amid fears the virus rises sharply, which could be spread by human contact with millions of Asians traveling for the holidays Lunar New Year this week. In China, the number of confirmed cases rose to 291 Monday.

CHAPTER 7: HOW TO THINK OF TRAVEL AS IT EVOLVES THE CORONAVIRUS THREAT

(Enisaurus for the Washington Post)

By Hannah Sampson March 2,

Travelers could quickly adapt in the early days of the outbreak of coronavirus when the disease was contained mainly a province in China. Then they began to appear cases and spread in other countries.

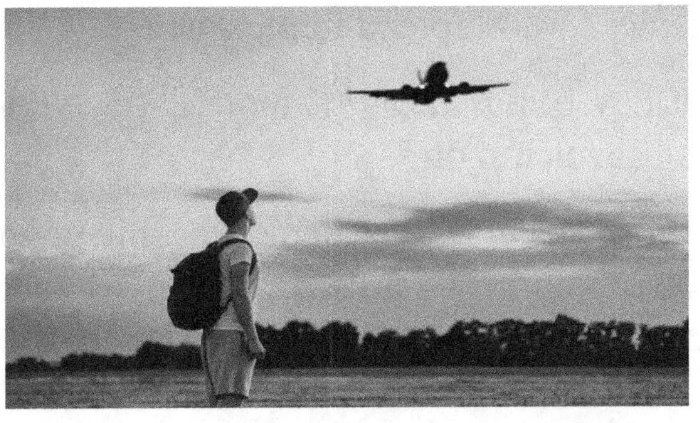

Concerns about the widespread disease in places like Italy anxieties brought closer to American travelers. Friday night, the U.S. State Department raised its warning level to warn Americans to reconsider travel throughout Italy due to "sustained community spread" of the virus. He warned not to travel in the regions of Lombardy and Veneto. More than 1,600 people have tested positive there. The Centers for Disease Control and Disease Prevention also raised its tongue over the country, issuing a warning to avoid all non-essential travel.

"I would not be predicted a week ago that northern Italy would be a place that can not travel at the moment would," Robert Quigley, regional medical director for risk mitigation travel company International SOS, said Thursday before warnings were lifted. "You can not predict where will be the next success."

Last week, authorities confirmed cases in the United States without known origin, which marks a new chapter for the spread in the country.

As each day brings news of more cases, which is a potential traveler to do?

Is it time to cancel a trip? Should people get on with their holiday and programadas-? And for those who still determined to travel, what is the best way to plan?

If you decide to cancel

Stay on the site is not a common practice in the past few days. Large corporations suspended large gatherings, and hotel chains reported increasing cancellations. Some travel agents say customers are canceling plans cruises abroad and changing US-based outputs or all-inclusive resorts. Like American Airlines, JetBlue and Alaska, waived cancellation and change fees for new customer bookings case get nervous about traveling.

Experts say there are potential resources. Travelers should consider deciding whether to call off a trip, including counseling and situation reports from the World Health Organization, warnings of the State Department, which often contain detailed information about specific regions within a country and communications CDC. From Monday the Food and Drug Administration warned the non-essential American travel to China, Iran, South Korea, and Italy, and improve the protection measures in Japan due to the corona to be avoided.

Few people are March 2 in Piazza Navona in Rome, which is usually full of tourists. Italy's tourism industry has been affected by the coronavirus outbreak, with hotel-reporting cancellations in droves, even in cities with few or no cases of the virus. (Remo Casilli / Reuters)

"I think right now, we see that more transmission in certain parts of the world, and so it is important to keep in mind where it was reported to transfer," said Crystal Watson, an assistant professor at Johns Hopkins University Center for Health, safety."Those places might not be the best places to go if you can avoid traveling there. But I that soon we will see a lot more transmission worldwide."

CHAPTER 8: THESE AIRLINES OFFER FLEXIBLE TRAVEL OPTIONS, ADAPT TO THE SPREAD OF THE CORONA.

To choose those who know what to do, said Watson should consider whether they are at a higher risk of serious illness if infected. This includes people over 65 and those with underlying health conditions.

Isaac Bogoch, an infectious disease physician and scientist at the University of Toronto, said that although the patterns so far show most people infected with coronavirus have mild symptoms, there are still many questions.

"I think we have to stay still modest as we do not have the answers," he said. "Because of this and because we do not have a vaccine and because we do not know a lot about this virus, people can have some fear wherever there are unknowns. "

Square mouth, the travel insurance comparison site, noted a "huge spike" in customer calls last week after the virus spread in Italy. According to a company survey offers, after people buy insurance, 27 percent said they purchased because of the coronavirus.

"Right now, we hear mainly customers who want to cancel their trip because they are worried about how the virus will spread, while the general feeling of fear and uncertainty," said the spokesman mouth square Kasara Barto. "Or they are still planning to travel, but they want to be able to buy a policy that allows them to cancel in case the epidemic spreads. "

Companies canceling U.S. domestic travel on fears coronavirus

Most booked and want to cancel because they are afraid to travel or because their primary reason for traveling may not be valid. They would be out of luck unless they purchased a comprehensive policy that allows them to call their travel for any reason.

Barto recommends calling hotels, airlines, and cruise lines to see if they can waive rebooking fees, change travel dates, or offer flexibility. Those who have booked a trip with a travel agent must consider whether this person can have ongoing relationships with travel companies can help make changes without penalty, Becky Powell, President of the Pro-Travel International,

Laurel Brunvoll, the owner of Unforgettable Voyages travel agency, recommends taking a wait and see approach to the cancellation of know how the situation plays out.

"For areas with increased risk, while this may depend on when someone is planning to travel there,"

If you go ahead with a trip

Perhaps it would be too expensive to cancel. Maybe that travelers will not just reschedule, they are not in a high-risk group, and the destination is not under aboard. Whatever the reason, the trip is still on the table.

'Experts say the key before going to prepare in case the situation changes'

"I think if you are going to travel and I do not say this is a bad idea, I would like to take a vacation myself, I think people should be aware that there is a possibility that you might get stuck somewhere for a long time, "said Watson.

CHAPTER 9: WHAT YOU NEED TO KNOW ABOUT CORONAVIRUSES

Bc coronavirus has made Italy a level 3 "do not travel if you can help" area myself. My sister and my mother called to see where we can go instead of Italy lol.

March 1, 2020

She said during a trip, and travelers should monitor new changes and adjust their behavior accordingly if the disease runs in a community staying away from public places, anyone who appears sick and large gatherings of people.

Some countries restrict where people can go or if someone is allowed into the affected areas, which could interfere with travel plans. Popular attractions may not be open; Louvre closed on Sunday and the Disney theme parks in Shanghai, Hong Kong, and Tokyo while temporarily closed.

A sign informs people about the closure of the Louvre Museum in Paris, March 2 (Adrienne SURPRISE-Nant / Bloomberg News)

Tony Rocca-forte, the chief adviser of security at the World risk management company Aware, said in an email that travelers must build redundancy into their plans, adding the time delays and preparing to improvise if conditions change.

"Make backups of your backups for all your communication devices, batteries, food/water, medication/eyeglasses, financial tools, transportation, lodging, plane tickets, etc. ", he said.

Before leaving, he said, vacationers should get all their ducks in a house behind the line: update their wills and powers of attorney, confirm the life insurance and health insurance and update their International file vaccination. Travelers should create a detailed itinerary of where they will be and when to give a colleague or a trusted person at home.

What are the chances that you get sick of being on a plane?

Erika Richter, the spokesman for the American Society of Travel Advisors, said in an email that travelers might consider putting the work equipment with them in case they end up marooned and should bring extra copies of passport, itinerary and proof of insurance.

Watson said the recommendation is that people have 30 days of prescription drugs with them, and they should also bring their original prescription in case they need more on the road.

Anyone who is sick should not travel not only to avoid spreading the disease but also to prevent being pulled out of line and potentially quarantined, said Quigley, International SOS.

He said carefully wipe the moving surfaces is "always in order," because many viruses and bacteria can survive on objects. The CDC said it might be possible for a person to get the coronavirus by touching something that has the virus and then touching your mouth, nose, or eyes, but it is not yet known how long the virus can survive on surfaces.

The bases are crucial to prevent infection, Courtney Kansler, senior health information analyst world Aware.

"This frequently includes with soap hand washing and water or use a sanitizer alcohol-based hand rub if soap and water are not available," she said. "Use social distancing and avoiding sick people. Transit quickly in airports and transportation hubs in the same crowded. "

Travelers who had not bought travel insurance when they booked a trip should consider adding a medical policy before going out, Barto square mouth said that the coverage is limited. She said last week that nearly a third of suppliers on the site offer coverage that would include the virus.

I am genuinely concerned about the coronavirus, but I'm also worried about the insane amount of money that my mother and I will not return if travel is entirely closed in the following month.

Jacqueline February 28, 2020

If you see the future Travel

For some travelers, no virus spread will be enough to stifle Wanderlust, especially with spring break and the season of the summer holiday approaches.

So how to proceed?

There are travel advisories and official warnings about where not to go. And the maps show where the spread of the virus. But experts warn against simply choose a place that has not seen a confirmed case.

"Every day we see reports of an increasing number of countries its first cases of the virus, and in addition to this, we see the countries known to have the virus report an increase," Bogoch said, the specialist in infectious diseases research co-author in the spread of the virus."If we are not calling this pandemic, at least we are sitting on the precipice of an epidemic. "

Quigley said it is essential for travelers always to look to be applied regulations and rules wherever they go and achieve everything that could change if and when the World Health Organization declared a pandemic.

"The answers everything will be different, but there will be a significant impact on both domestic travel and across borders," he said.

Travelers considering where to go potential consequences need factors for the spread of the virus' in their decision-making, Rocca-forte said, of the world is aware. He said that includes the possibility of quarantines, travel restrictions, bans on public transport, water and food rationing, social unrest, and strained health systems.

Anyone traveling should think about what they would find medical attention if pain or sick.

"This is more important for people who have underlying health problems, and becomes even more important if an infectious disease outbreak occurs," Watson said the Johns Hopkins Center for Health Safety.

Making those plans now can still buy insurance if they decide after canceling due to fears of coronavirus, but the policy will not be cheap.

"Right now, the only and best option we recommend for people is a 'cancel for any reason' policy," Barto said. He said that which is only available within the first 10 to 21 days of booking a trip costs about 40 percent more than standard cancellation policy. It reimburses 75 percent of the cost of the trip.

Richter, the spokesman for the American Society of Travel Advisors, suggests using a professional to help make plans for spring or summer.

"A travel consultant can help you through your list of options and prices that can help you come up with a plan A, B, and C and have those options backup on hand talk can put your mind at ease.

"In times like these, a defender of travel is required."

Economic forecasts
global growth

The financial situation remains very fluid. Uncertainty about the duration and depth of the economic effects of the health crisis fuels the perception of risk and volatility in financial markets and corporate decision-making. Also, doubts about the global pandemic and effectiveness of public policies to limit its spread add to the volatility of the market.

Compounding the economic situation is a historic fall in the price of crude oil, reflecting the overall decline in economic activity prospects for disinflation. It contributes to the deterioration of the global economy through various channels. On April 29, 2020, Federal Reserve Chairman Jay Powell said the Federal Reserve could use its "full range of tools" to support economic activity as the Commerce Department reported a 4.8% drop in GDP EE .S. in the first quarter of 2020. was assessing the state of the U.S. economy, the Federal Open Market Committee issued a statement saying that "public health crisis underway in the short term and poses profoundly on economic activity, employment and inflation burden significant risks to the economic outlook in the medium term. "

The Organization for Economic Co-operation and Development (OECD), on March 2, 2020, I reduced its forecast for global economic growth at 0.5% for 2020 from 2.9% to 2.4%, based on the assumption that the economic effects of the virus would peak in the first quarter of 202016. However, the OECD estimates that if the economic impact of the disease does not arise in the first quarter, it is now clear that it was not, global economic growth would increase by 1.5% in 2020. this forecast seems now to have been very optimistic.

On March 23, 2020, the Secretary-General of the OECD, Angel Gurria, said:

The magnitude of the current shock introduces unprecedented complexity for economic forecasting. The Interim Economic Outlook OECD, published on March 2, 2020, made the first attempt to take stock of the likely impact of COVID-19 on global growth. Still, it seems that we have moved beyond even the most severe scenario than expected pandemic. It has also launched a major economic crisis that will burden our societies in the coming years.

On March 26, 2020, the OECD revised its global economic forecast based on the continuing effects of the pandemic, and governments have adopted measures to contain the spread of the virus. According to the updated estimate, measures current containment could reduce global GDP of 2.0% per month, or an annual rate of 24%, approaching the level of economic contraction not experienced since the Great Depression of the decade 1930. the OECD estimates will be revised when the OECD releases updated data specific to the country.

Labeling the expected decline in global economic activity as the "Great Lockdown," the IMF released a forecast updated on April 14, 2020. The IMF concluded that the global economy could experience its "worst recession since the Great Depression, beating observed during the Global financial crisis a decade "The IMF estimated that the worldwide economy could decline by 3.0% in 2020 before growing by 5.8% in 2021 ago, it is expected that world trade to fall in 2020 11.0% and is expected to oil prices falling by 42%.

This assumes that the prognosis pandemic fades in the second half of 2020 and that containment measures can be reversed quickly.

The IMF also noted that many countries face multiple layers, including a health crisis, an internal economic crisis, a fall in external demand, capital outflows, and a fall in raw materials prices. In combination, these various effects are interacting in ways that make the prediction difficult.

Are advanced forecast economies as a group to experience an economic contraction in 2020 of 7.8% of GDP, with the U.S. economy by the IMF projected to decline by 5.9%, almost twice the rate decline experienced in 2009 during the financial crisis, as indicated. The price of economic growth in the eurozone is expected to decline by 7.5% of GDP. It is anticipated that most developing economies and emerging experience a decrease in the rate of economic growth of 2.0%, reflecting the tightening of global financial conditions and falling prices trade and commodities throughout the world. By contrast, China, India, and Indonesia are expected to experience low but favorable economic growth rates in 2020. The IMF also argues that the recovery of the global economy could be weaker than expected due to persistent uncertainty on a possible contagion, lack of confidence, and the permanent closure of companies and changes in companies and households.

Before the COVID-19 pop, the world economy was struggling to regain a broad-based recovery as a result of the continuing impact of rising trade protectionism, trade disputes between major trading partners, falling prices of raw materials and energy, and economic uncertainty in Europe over the effect of the withdrawal of the U.K. from the European Union. Individually, each of these topics presented a solvable challenge for the world economy. Altogether, however, the problems weakened the global economy and reducing the policy flexibility of many national leaders, especially among the major developed economies available. In this environment, COVID-19.

You could have a considerable impact. While the level of economic effects over time becomes more explicit, the response to the pandemic could have a significant effect and last in the way companies organize their workforces, global supply chains, and how governments respond to a health crisis worldwide.

The OECD estimates that direct and indirect economic costs increased by global supply chains. The demand for goods and services and lower tourist and business trips decreased mean that "the negative consequences of these developments in other countries (non-OECD) are important." World trade measured by trading volume slowed in the last quarter of 2019 and is expected in 2020 related to the pandemic due to the weaker global economy are declining, in different areas harms economic activity, including airlines, hospitality, sports, and marine industry.

According to OECD forecasts updated:

The most significant impact confinement restrictions will be on retail and wholesale trade, professional services, and real estate, although there are substantial differences between countries.

closures could reduce economic output in advanced countries and major emerging economies by 15% or more; other emerging economies could experience a drop in production of 25%.

countries that depend on tourism could be affected more severely, while countries with agricultural and mining sectors could suffer less severe effects.

The economic impacts are likely to vary between countries reflect differences in the timing and degree of containment measures.

Also, the OECD says that China's emergence as a global economic player marks a significant departure from previous comprehensive health episodes. China's growth, combined with globalization and interdependence of economies through capital flows, supply chains, and foreign investment, magnifies the cost of the spread of the virus through quarantines and restricted mobility of labor and travel.

The global economic role of China and globalization mean that trade plays a role in the dissemination of economic effects Covid-19.

More generally, the economic impact of the pandemic spreads through three sales channels:

1. by supply chains that the reduced economic activity covered by producers of intermediate goods to finished goods producers.
2. due to an overall decline in economic activity, reducing demand for products in general, including imports.
3. by reduced trade with commodity exporters that supply producers, who, in turn, reduced their imports and negatively affects the trade and economic activity of the exporters.

Global trade

By April 8, 2020, provided by the World Trade Organization (WTO), it is expected that the volume of world trade will decline between 13% and 32% by 2020 as a result of the economic impact of COVID-19, WTO, as shown in Table 2, found the entire spectrum of the high level of uncertainty in forecasting the Treasury in terms of duration and economic impact of the pandemic and actual is outside this range could result, and more upper or lower.

Most optimistic scenario assumes that WTO trade volumes recover quickly in the second half of 2020 to its previous trend pandemic, or that the world economy is recovering as V. The most pessimistic scenario assumes a partial recovery which lasts until 2021 or suffering from the global economic activity over improvement in the form of U. The WTO concluded that the impact on the volume of world trade could surpass the fall of world trade during the height of the financial crisis of 2008-2009.

Estimates show that all geographic regions will experience a decline in the double-digit trading volume for "other regions," which from Africa, the Middle East, and the Commonwealth of Independent States with the exception. North America and Asia would experience the most significant declines in export volumes. The forecast also projects that sectors with high-value chains such as automotive products and electronics could suffer the most significant reductions.

Although services are not included in the forecast of the WTO, this segment of the economy could suffer the most significant changes as a result of restrictions on travel and transport and closing commercial establishments and hospitality. However, services such as information technology are growing to meet the demand of employees working from home.

Economic policy challenges

The challenge for the authorities has been implementing specific policies to deal with the expected short-term problems without creating distortions in the economy that survive the virus's effects. However, policymakers are being overtaken by the rapidly changing nature of the global health crisis that seems to be becoming a world trade and the economic crisis, whose effects on the economy worldwide are increasing.

As the economic impact of the pandemic grows, the authorities are giving more weight to policies that address the immediate financial consequences at the expense of long-term considerations, such as debt accumulation. Initially, many politicians had felt limited To respond in their ability the crisis as a result of the limited flexibility of monetary and fiscal support in conventional standards, given the synchronized slowdown broad-based global economic growth, particularly in the manufacture and trade that had developed viral outbreak.

The pandemic is also affecting global politics, and global leaders are canceling international meetings28, and some nations.

According to reports, they are fueling conspiracy theories that blame other countries.

Initially, it was expected that the economic effects of the virus to be Supply problems in the short term as a factory were issued because workers were to reduce the spread of the virus through social interaction quarantined.

The decline in economic activity, initially in China, has had international repercussions as companies experienced delays in deliveries of intermediate and finished goods through the supply chain.

Raise concerns, however, that the supply shock related virus is creating demand shocks longer and far-reaching as reduced activity by consumers and businesses have a lower rate of economic growth. As demand shocks are developed, companies are experiencing reduced activity, increased benefits, and potentially binding credit constraints and liquidity.

While manufacturing companies are experiencing crashes and supply chains, reduced consumer activity through social distancing affects the service sector of the economy, accounting for two-thirds of

the U.S. annual economic output. In this environment, manufacturing and service companies have tended to treasure money in cash, which affects market liquidity. In response, central banks have cut interest rates when possible and extended loan services to provide liquidity to financial markets and the company may be insolvent.

The longer the economic impact is made, the higher the economic impact should the results be transferred from commercial and financial relations with an ever-larger group of countries, companies, and households. Potentially increase this growing economic impact of liquidity constraints and credit market in the global financial markets attracting businesses to accumulate cash, with adverse effects on economic growth fallout. At the same time, the financial markets to an increase in bond issuance by the Government of factoringUnited States, Europe, and other places such as public debt levels increased to meet expected spending obligations during an economic downturn expected to increase.

Fiscal spending to combat the effects of the COVID-19.

Unlike the 2008-2009 financial crisis, reduced consumer demand, labor market issues, and a lower level of activity among enterprises,

instead of risky trading by banks worldwide, led to corporate credit problems and potential bankruptcy. These market dynamics have led some observers to question whether these events Scale Full-financial crisis marks the beginning of a global.

Market liquidity and credit policy questions were several different challenges to face supply shortages. As a result, the focus has government policy has expandable from a health crisis to the problems of macroeconomic and financial market through a combination of monetary, fiscal, and others, including border closures, quarantines, and restrictions on social interactions.

In essence, while businesses are trying to worker issues and address output at the company level, national leaders are trying to implement fiscal policies to prevent economic growth fell sharply for helping workers and businesses facing economic tensions, and central banks are adapting monetary policy to the problems of the credit market steering assembly.

In the initial phase of the health, crisis households experienced not the same kind of loss of wealth, which they saw during the financial crisis of 2008-2009 when the value of their primary residence drastically reduced. However, with numbers rapidly increasing unemployment, job losses could lead to mortgage defaults and delinquencies in payment of rent, unless financial institutions provide loan tolerance or a mechanism to provide financial assistance. In turn, the mortgage defaults could adversely affect the market for mortgage-backed securities, the availability of mortgage funds, and negatively affect the overall rate of economic growth. Losses in the value of most stock markets in the US, Asia, and Europe could also affect household wealth, especially retirees living on a fixed income and others who own shares.

Investors trading mortgage-backed securities reports have been reducing their holdings while the Federal Reserve has been trying to support it.31 In the current environment, including traditional policy instruments such as monetary accommodation at the seem, have not been conventionally processed by the markets, with indices of the stock market Displaying increased, rather than the lower levels, uncertainty after the Federal Reserve cut interest rates, the volatility Such is adding to doubts about what governments can do to address deficiencies in the global economy.

Economic Developments

Between late February and April 2020, the financial markets of the United States to Asia and Europe have already been whipsawed investors have grown concerned that COVID-19 would create the economic and financial crisis overall with indicators to indicate how long and extensive economic effects can be.32 investors searched for investment haven, as the benchmark U.S. Treasury security ten years, experienced a record drop in yield below 1%, March

3 2020.33 in response to concerns that the global economy was in a freefall, the Fed reduced interest rates on March 3, 2020, to support economic activity, while the Bank of Japan spent on shopping assets to provide short-term liquidity to Japanese banks; The Government of Japan indicated that it would also help workers with wage subsidies.

The Bank of Canada also cut its first interest rate. The International Monetary Fund (IMF) announced that it was about $ 50 trillion available through emergency financing facilities for low-income and emerging countries and funds available through its containment disaster and relief Trust (CCRT).

The uncertainty of investors, the Dow Jones Industrial Average (DJIA) lost equivalent to about a third of its value between February 14, 2020, and March 23, 2020, the expectation that the U.S. Congress could be a package of $ 2.0 trillion spending Dow Jones will have shifted by more than 11% on March 24, 2020 move from March 23 to April 15 Dow Jones higher by18%. Since then, the Dow Jones has moved erratically as investors weighed news about the human cost and economic impact of the pandemic and prospects of various medical treatments. For some politicians, the fall in stock prices has raised concerns that foreign investors could try to take advantage of the situation by increasing the purchases of companies in sectors that are considered national security as necessary. Ursula von der Leyen, President of the European Commission, called for E.U.. members to better screen foreign investment, especially in areas such as health, medical research, and infrastructure.35 similar criticism to the global financial crisis of 2008-2009, the central banks have implemented several monetary transactions to provide liquidity to their economies.

These actions, however, were initially not entirely positive by all participants in the financial market that questioned the use of policy instruments of central banks, which are similar to those employed during the financial crisis of 2008-2009, despite the current crisis this is fundamentally different in origin.

In the last financial crisis, central banks intervened to restart lending and spending of banks that had participated in risky assets. In the current environment, central banks are trying to cope with the volatility of the financial market and prevent large-scale reflect underlying economic uncertainty caused by the pandemic business insolvencies.

A the same as in the conditions during the financial crisis of 2008-2009, the dollar has become the preferred currency by investors, reinforcing its role as a dominant reserve currency world, the dollar rose more than 3.0% during the period March 3y 13,

2020, reflecting the increase in international demand for the dollar and dollar-denominated assets. From their highs on March 23, the dollar has given up some of its value against other currencies but has remained around 10% higher than it was at the beginning of the year.

A recent survey conducted by the Bank for International Settlements (BIS) represents $ 36 for 88% of the global turnover of the foreign exchange market. It is crucial in financing a series of financial transactions, including serving as an invoicing currency to facilitate international trade. It also represents two-thirds of foreign exchange reserves of central banks, half of the foreign currency deposits of the non-US bank, and two-thirds of non-US corporate loans from banks and corporate bond markets.37 As a result, interruptions in the functioning of the world market for the dollar may have a far-reaching impact on international trade and financial proceedings.

The international role of the dollar also increases the pressure on the Federal Reserve to necessarily assume the lead role as a global lender of last resort. Reminiscent of the financial crisis, the world economy has experienced a period of shortage of dollars, requiring the Federal Reserve to take numerous measures to ensure the supply of dollars to the U.S. and global economies, including activation of existing currency swap contracts, the establishment of such new agreements with central banks, and the creation of new financial services to provide liquidity to central banks

monetary authorities.38 Generally, banks lend long-term and short-term loan and can only borrow from their local central bank. In turn, central banks can only provide liquidity in the currency.

Consequently, a bank can not cash in a panic, which means that it can borrow in private markets to meet cash flow needs in the short term. Swap lines are designed to allow foreign central banks to provide the necessary liquidity to banks in their country in dollars.

The bond yields of the U.S. Treasury fell to historic lows on March 6, 2020. March 9, 2020, as investors continue to move out of stocks and securities of the Treasury and other government securities, including the U.K. and German bonds were due to concerns about the impact of the pandemic in part on the growth and economic expectations that the Federal Reserve and other central banks short-term interest rates.39 could cut on March 5, U.S. Congress approved an expenditure of $ 8Billion bills to health aid, sick, small business loans and international cooperation. At the same time, prices of raw materials declined sharply as a result of reduced economic activity and disagreements among producers of more cuts oil production of crude oil and lower global demand for commodities, including oil raw.

CONCLUSION

This book explains about the world situation and the impact based on the global economy on Covid-19, teach us the skills on how to use a face mask and describe and list how to make a face mask in different type with a simple step to protect and give information about social boost, the impact it has had on tourism and the situation in travel and holidays.